SHE COMES FIRST

Strategies of the high-value woman

A book about standing your ground in dating, in marriage, in your career, and everywhere else!

Disclaimer

The Elephant in the Room

Let's start off by addressing the obnoxious elephant in the room. You're about to read a book about female empowerment, written by a man. Yes, I know, there are weirder things in life. But still, I can imagine you have a sense that something is amiss.

I've been coaching women in their love lives for over a decade and have written a couple of bestsellers in the marriage and love and dating categories. I can do that because, as a man, I know a lot of counterintuitive facts about men and their behavior. As I was coaching women and helping them in their relationships, I began to unravel something bigger than even their love lives. Something huge. I noticed a lot of these ladies had problems with *being* women.

They weren't totally fulfilled. Not just in their relationships, but in life. Some had unfulfilling jobs, didn't get paid what they were worth, had always dreamt of starting their own business but never did, felt lonely even though they had a husband and kids... the list goes on and on. Some women had everything they could desire but *still* felt that something was missing.

So many women try to be the perfect girlfriends, wives, mothers, friends, sisters, colleagues, business owners, bosses, and more. They love to serve and want to succeed in the many roles they have to play. They are compliant, even to the people who don't really deserve that kind of treatment. They give it all they have, every single day.

Regardless of their tremendous efforts, some women get little in return. They feel used. They get men that keep flaking out, careers that don't feel meaningful, and possibly a body that starts to feel and look more and more tired. Did you ever notice that burnouts tend to afflict women much more often than men? There's a reason for that, as you'll learn.

This should stop.

Some of these women wonder if they should just readjust their expectations and conform to what society has told them their role and behavior should be like.

Maybe they should accept that their relationship or marriage is becoming as passionless and cold as your average Siberian winter.

Maybe they should accept that their professional lives make them feel bored, burnt out, or frustrated.

Maybe they should accept that they have to push aside their own dreams and goals so they can care for others.

When they do, these women start to believe *they* are the problem. Let me assure you, they are not. It's not their fault.

I've been writing books for women for many years now because I can't take it anymore. Women deserve better! *You* deserve better.

There's something misaligned in society today: some women are not allowing themselves to reach their full potential—to be everything they are meant to be. They keep themselves small for reasons that we'll explore throughout the book.

Women have *more* on their plates than ever before in the history of womankind.
They try to juggle their careers while finding and keeping a great partner, maybe raising some kids and a goldfish, and doing

household chores. They do this while looking put together and while trying to remain physically fit and radiant—almost as if somebody is continuously photoshopping them.

I'm even getting tired just thinking about the workload most women face.

Nevertheless, some women seem to have found a loophole, a backdoor in the current system. There are women out there who have designed the life they live. I call these women the high-value women.

This value has nothing to do with money. The high-value woman knows very well what she wants, and most of the time, she gets it too. Boredom, burnout, depression, and even chronic frustration are not in her dictionary. I've been studying and interviewing this type of woman for more than a decade now, trying to figure out how she does it. Through careful research and important conversations with many different high-value women, I discovered the common denominators.

It turns out the high-value woman follows a set of strategies and principles. I'll share them with you throughout this book.

 You might have seen and met her. She's the woman who is self-employed, doing the thing she loves and making a living off of it. She's the woman who might have decided to have a normal career, with a twist. It's the type of career she enjoys, and she is actually appreciated for the hard work and hours she puts into it.

When she speaks, others listen, *even* the men in her office with overinflated egos. Her job almost never feels like work and is deeply fulfilling. It doesn't cost her energy; she *gets* energy from it. When she wakes up, she can't wait to get started with her day.

She is the woman who has found and created herself a loving relationship with a man she loves. Their relationship is based on mutual respect, equality, affection, passion, and true friendship. They operate as a great team, and tasks and responsibilities are equally shared. She has this type of relationship because she would have never settled for anything less. Her list of "things I want to change about him" is rather short or nonexistent.

She is *also* the woman who is happily single, the woman who doesn't *need* a man to be happy. She has a supportive circle of great friends, and she has the time to hang out with them, *even* when she has kids. She knows how to set the world to *her* hand, so it seems, and some women wonder how she does it.

However, when you look more closely, you'll find out she's not a magician—she doesn't have any special powers. She simply knows how to tap into the power that every woman has. Some women have just forgotten how to use that strength.

I call that power the lioness.

I could have used spiritual words like goddess or warrior—but what we're about to embark upon is not really spiritual. We're going to build on scientific research and feedback from the real world. The strategies that you'll discover have been tested in real life. And they really work.

As a reminder, using your power isn't about getting rich, indulging in spiritual stuff, becoming the next president or the prettiest woman alive. Far from it. A powerful high-value woman uses her internal strength, her emotional intelligence, and all of the resources available to her to design and craft the life she really wants to live. She doesn't hold back. She doesn't adapt nor does she try to please anyone. She's her own authentic self most of the time, if not all of the time.

She can be pretty, average, or even downright hard to look at. She can be athletic, thin, overweight. She can be rich, middle-class, or poor. It doesn't matter where she stands on all of these ladders; she feels content; she doesn't lack anything. She loves her life and in return, life seems to love her back.

This book is not about becoming someone you're not. It's about becoming who you *are.* This book is about you. It's about your empowerment, about taking back what's yours.

We'll dive into your romantic relationships, your career, your personal life, and most importantly, your own mind.

I'm sure you already are a high-value woman in many ways. Some parts of the book will reaffirm that you're on the right track; others will provide a new way of thinking to take you to the next level.

Are you curious to find out how the high-value woman does it all?

Let's go!

Brian

The Scripts of Life You Pick

Most people prefer to continue doing what they have always been doing, living day in and day out using the same scripts over and over again. To them, life is one huge repetition of habits.

And they may not even be their own habits and scripts. As they were growing up, they got a lot of important life lessons from well-meaning people who always knew better and they have based parts of their life upon them. Nevertheless, these lessons didn't always represent the truth.

Do any of these sound familiar?

"No, you're not supposed to do that!"

Instead of

"Truth be told, you really should go after what you want. I wish I had. But I can't tell you that because then I will feel like a failure myself."

"Still single? A girl like you should be able to find a boyfriend, shouldn't you?"

Instead of

"Men don't make sense to me. Do not, under any circumstances, take my advice on men. You may have noticed how unhappy I am with your uncle. I wish I were single, like you. But I can't tell you that. I would lose my position as your all-knowing auntie, and that's all I've got going for me."

"Becoming self-employed in *this* economy? You crazy?"

Instead of

"Truth be told, I got fired last week after working my ass off for twenty years. I had so many great ideas to venture out on my own, but I never did. I hope you don't either because that's going to be hard for me to accept..."

And there you were, thinking the lies were over after you found out Santa and the Easter Bunny aren't real. It never ceases to amaze me what people have kept feeding us just because they thought it was in our (um, their) best interest.

Some people are stuck in the scripts they have been forced into, and their life is zooming by. They complain about the same problems over and over again, and they're not getting ahead. They keep chasing the same dreams—often in the wrong way— and they feel like everything they really want is unreachable. It's not meant for them, apparently.

You are different; otherwise, you wouldn't have picked up this book. I'm sure you are already succeeding well in many areas of life where you are getting great results.

On the other hand, because you are a woman, you've also felt the need to put others first, to find a good work-life balance, to be a good girlfriend/wife/mother/friend, to have the perfect body, to keep up with the Joneses, etc. It's a need that partially comes from within you, but the media and especially *social* media play a much bigger role and continue to dictate how you are supposed to live your life too.

How do you *really* feel when you scroll through your social media feed? I bet it feels like you're missing out on a lot. Or at least that other people seem to have it all figured out much better than you. There they are, having perfect friends, perfect skin, and perfect experiences. They are living superior lives in a perpetual state of happiness that even feel-good movies have a hard time portraying. They seem to have experiences and states of happiness that elude most of us. You may start to feel a gap between where you are in life and where everyone else seems to be living.

You are not alone!

And for a lot of people, this creates feelings of emptiness that they try to fill. Some pick healthy strategies like doing yoga, meditation, sipping green drinks, working out, trying to find love, making babies, going for that great career, and often all of the above combined. Others pick the dark side and go for food with excessive sugar, bad fats, shopping sprees, or even bad relationships that keep them busy—*very* busy—all in an effort to ignore the feeling that something is missing.

Nevertheless, this hunger cannot be satisfied with things. It can't even be appeased by boyfriends, husbands, babies, or the cutest kitty cat. So many women are convinced they need to have a boyfriend or husband, have babies, have this or that, and *then* everything will be all right. It won't, as many of them find out time and time again.

When I look at all of the high-value women I've interviewed, I notice that they know who they are and what they want. Some want to have a great relationship and get it; others prefer to be single and love it. Some want to start a family and do; others have decided they don't want kids and are totally fine too.

The big difference is these were all 100 percent their own decisions. They don't follow a prewritten script of life, they write their own. They are little to not influenced by society and do what feels good to *them,* most of the time.

But the reason why they can satisfy that hunger is that they follow a different strategy compared to the masses. High-value women have woken up. They are not in reaction-mode, just taking in what happens to come along. They go after what they want. They are very aware of how negative emotions, self-limiting beliefs, and even the blatant lies of society are trying to hinder their growth, and they know exactly how to deal with it all.

High-value women live a life driven more by curiosity than fear.

Most importantly, they are not trying to dismiss or avoid negative emotions. Instead, they are putting their energy toward going after what they want.

Of course, the road to fulfillment is covered with obstacles. We will go over how to deal with those in what follows.

Strapped Down Nice and Tight

When a woman loses touch with her inner lioness, she starts to suffer from a variety of feelings and emotions, as if her soul is being strangled. It is! It's being strapped down, nice and tight, barely able to breathe and survive. The woman in question is deviating from what makes her truly alive and happy.

This has consequences. She can suffer from fatigue, disinterest, burnout, boredom, depression, loss of passion, emotional instability, loss of identity, feelings of helplessness and powerlessness, and worst of all, she can start to feel weak and needy *even though she is a strong woman*. She will have thoughts like "I'm normally not like this" or "I used to be different."

Needless to say, it's important to avoid this.

The question is, when do you strangle your soul? It happens when you ignore it. Most women have already noticed there is a part of themselves they have not yet fully tapped into. Maybe they did for a while until life's circumstances took over. Some women fantasize about what that suppressed part of them wants. Nevertheless, most are afraid to do something about it.

Some of the bondage and soul-tying is brought upon us by ourselves. Many of our limitations are self-imposed because we keep believing them, even though deep down we know they may not be accurate. Some examples include:

- "I need to be in a relationship to be someone."
- "I need to be at my ideal weight to be happy."
- "My skin needs to look perfect; otherwise, I'm not attractive."
- "I need to always be willing to help and serve; otherwise, I'm not a good girlfriend/wife/mother/friend."

- "I'm not beautiful or smart enough to..."
- "Now is not the right time in my life to..."
- "First I need to ... and then I will finally be able to..."

Wait a minute! These are only true if we decide they are! That's why these are called *self*-limiting beliefs.

On the other hand, some women domesticate their dreams and aspirations because everyone else seems to be instructing them to do just that. Some well-meaning friends and family say, "Are you *sure* that's a good idea? I wouldn't do it!" whenever you dream out loud. Some aggressive and competitive friends or co-workers may love to give unconstructive criticism even though you didn't ask for it.

The media plays a role here too, with some magazine covers screaming:

- "What guys hate for you to wear in bed" (Um, a clown costume maybe?)
- "Be the best lover on your block" (Good luck with *that!*)
- "What he wants to see during sex" (*Games of Thrones*? *Jurassic Park*? No idea really...)

while portraying photoshopped women, upholding an ideal impossible to attain. These covers and the related articles often imply that who you are now is not enough. Needless to say, some men's magazines are no different.

The fact that the media influences us has not only been scientifically proven, it's the very reason why we consume it. When you watch your favorite TV show or buy a magazine, you're not just killing time. You do it because it gives you feelings, because it influences you in some way. Social psychology professor Karen Dill even proved that the world of fiction and the media as a whole can change our belief system and ideas.[1]

We are getting examples of how we are supposed to be living our lives everywhere around us, and we are continuously reminded of what society's standards are and what track we should adhere to. Success is often portrayed as: make a lot of money, get a great relationship, have the perfect body/skin/weight, feel emotionally well all the time, do not show signs of aging, have perfect and happy kids, and don't have any flaws or shortcomings, at all. In short, if *this* is not what your life looks like, then you must not be doing it right.

How could you possibly *not* feel overwhelmed?

What feels right to us personally on the surface level *is* often dictated and heavily influenced by all of these forces around us. We may sometimes believe that something was our choice, when it really wasn't. Our egos love to believe that each choice we make is based upon our own individual judgement and independent assessment, but research proves that is simply not the case. Please let this sink in for a moment. Some of the choices we make in life are not our own. Even though we believe they are.

There are multiple scientific studies to prove it.[2] One of my favorites is the so-called coffee study performed by John A. Bargh, a professor at Yale University. In that simple experiment, people's judgements of a stranger were altered by handing that stranger a hot cup of coffee (as in, people felt more positive about a stranger with a hot cup of coffee than a stranger without

---

[1] Karen Dill, How Fantasy Becomes Reality: Seeing through Media Influence (2009), 224.
[2] Who's minding the Mind, Benedict Carey, July 31, 2007 – *The New York Times*

one). The reason why is interesting. On the way to the laboratory, the research participants had seemingly accidently bumped into a laboratory assistant who was holding textbooks, papers, a clipboard, and a hot coffee. This assistant then asked them for a hand by holding the cup. This small, manipulated event was all it took to influence the ratings the participants gave (those who weren't asked for a hand or got a *cold* cup of coffee rated the stranger differently). Other studies also proved that these almost subliminal "messages" we get influence our goals, our choices, and so much more through our subconscious brain.[3] Even the music we listen to while shopping influences what we buy and how much we're willing to pay for it, as a study that was presented by the Association of Psychological Science proves.[4] Long story short, even though we often love to believe we are immune to all of this, we really aren't. It always influences us to some extent.

With all of those outside influences impacting us, we need to be mindful. What about what YOU want and need specifically in the relationships you have, the career you pick, and what you spend your time on otherwise? What fulfills *you*? What about your many purposes here on Earth?

It's pretty pointless to keep running after goals that are indirectly imposed upon us when, deep down, we really don't care that much about achieving them. Given that happiness is most felt when we enjoy the journey and not just the destination, we need to make sure we are the ones picking the destination and the road to it.

---

[3] *The Unconscious Mind* - John A. Bargh and Ezequiel Morsella, 2008, https://www.ncbi.nlm.nih.gov/pmc/articles/PMC2440575/

[4] North, A. C., Sheridan, L. P., & Areni, C. S. (2015). Music Congruity Effects on Product Memory, Perception, and Choice. *Journal of Retailing.* doi:10.1016/j.jretai.2015.06.001

All of this explains why we are going to look behind all the noise and outside influences and get to what you really need and want. Because the answer to that question will be 100 percent unique to you.

To get to what you want and *really* need (not just on the surface level), you often need to dig a little bit deeper. But it's worth the effort. This life is not the dress rehearsal. This is the only life you get. This is *YOUR* life.

To arrive at what will make you deeply happy, we'll also need to discard everything that other people want from you to make *them* happy. Not so you can become an egocentric maniac who doesn't care about others but to see clearly, to lift the fog first.

It's OK to focus on what you want and need first. It's not selfish; it's crucial.

Just like the flight attendant always says, "When the oxygen masks drop from the cabin ceiling, please do not help children or others until you've securely attached the mask to yourself first." The reason why is interesting. If you faint due to a lack of oxygen, you won't be able to be of service to anyone else. You need to take care of yourself *first* in the event of an emergency.

I think that's a nice analogy for life. If you don't think of yourself first, you're no good to others anyway.

You come first.

The Price of "Yes"

Most women only need a couple of seconds to agree to help someone else. Be that a man they are dating, a husband, children, family members, even a boss or colleague. Heck, even their pets. They just want to do good and help out; the world is hard enough as it is.

It is seemingly effortless. But it comes at a really high price. You have a limited amount of energy and willpower every day, and when that energy supply is empty, the lights go out. When that happens, it becomes really hard to say "no" to everything you know you shouldn't do. Examples are declining that dessert you really shouldn't have, avoiding that text you really shouldn't send, or continuing to the "play the next episode" when you *really* shouldn't. The little traps of life become invisible. When the lights are out, there's nothing but darkness.

On top of that, the most precious resource you will ever own is time. No matter how poor or unbelievably rich you are, you can't buy more than twenty-four hours in a day. What you spend your time on counts.

When some women are asked to prioritize what is important to *them*, when they're asked what gives *them* joy, the answer is "I have no time for joy." And even if they do, they can't really enjoy it without feeling guilty. Something is always gnawing at the back of their minds.

There luckily is another way. Let's call it the way of the high-value woman.

Charlotte, a client of mine and a 37-year-old mother of two, was a great example of this predicament. She was a serious woman who had a flourishing career in advertising. Charlotte was making a significant amount of money, able to buy most of what she thought her heart desired. Her house had a pool, a sauna, and you would need a map when you entered her endless walk-in closet in order to find your way out. She was still able to drop off the kids at school every morning *and* prepare their lunch bags. The kids were raised well. Her husband was a good and kind guy too. They had nothing to complain about. The picture-perfect life from the outside, but the reality was quite different.

When Charlotte reached out she confided in me that she didn't know who she was. Her life was passing by quickly and although she was never bored and had *everything*, she told me, "I feel like I'm living every day on autopilot, taking care of problems and challenges in a never-ending loop. I never have time to enjoy any of it."

That wasn't all. Her sex life was virtually non-existent. She and her husband lived like brothers and sisters would. There was love, but the passion had vanished a long time ago. Charlotte and Kris, her husband, each had their own side on the couch and the line in the middle saw fewer crossings than a maximum security prison wall. No handholding, no passionate undressing with the soundtrack of *Basic Instinct* playing in the background. Nothing. Their sex life had tumbleweeds blowing through it.

All of her life, she had been of service to others. And not just when her first son was born. It started a lot earlier. Fresh out of college, she chased after success in advertising because she wanted to make her daddy proud. When she was dating her husband, she had begun to adapt to what was important to him. Not because Kris was a controlling dictator, but it was what she thought she was supposed to do. That's what her mother and other female role models had taught her.

There was a pivotal change when the kids were born. "I am a mother now," Charlotte thought. "I must always put them first and make sure that they get the best and most perfect upbringing possible." That's indeed a great formula to arrive in Boredom Ville. Ten years later, Charlotte had no real hobbies, no real passions—everything she did was to serve the needs of others. All of the passion projects and dreams she had when she was a teenager were gone, stored in a proverbial box hidden deep down somewhere in the attic with "For when I retire" written on it.

So many people are led to believe life starts when you retire. *Then* you'll have time to do the things *you* find important. Even a donkey wouldn't fall for that carrot on a stick. Yet I did too, for many years.

"Some people die at 25 but aren't buried until they are 75." Benjamin Franklin once said something similar, and he was spot on.[5]

Although Charlotte seemed a very serious and goal-oriented woman at first, I knew there was another girl hiding behind the mask and persona she had constructed so well. Charlotte had put aside her playful, confident, and feminine side to take on the role of serious mother and good wife, just like she was told to by her female peers.

It took me a while to make her see this, but as soon as the blinds had been removed and as soon as she began to implement what you will learn in the next chapters, Charlotte realized she could be a great mother and wife *and* take care of what was important to her.

---

[5] https://www.goodreads.com/quotes/993331-some-people-die-at-age-25-and-aren-t-buried-until

Long story short, she quit her advertising job and became a freelancing consultant. Now she picks her own hours. She created more time to spend on the things that mattered to her. Long walks alone in nature, taking a dance class with her husband, and finally learning how to play the piano (her lifelong dream) were only a couple of her new activities. The dance classes rekindled the flame between her and her husband. They even started to practice tantric bedroom games, just for fun. These are just some examples of the many changes that started to bring Charlotte in touch with her feminine energy, her lioness.

In stark contrast to what she had feared, her relationship with her kids benefitted, and they gave the feedback that they loved Mom 2.0.

Charlotte ditched most of the masculine energy she had been bathing herself in and embraced her feminine side to the fullest. She told me it made her feel alive, ecstatic even. For the first time in decades, she *loved* life again.

And as you'll see in many of the examples that follow, you don't even need to make the major changes Charlotte pushed through. Tiny one percent changes are often all that's needed.

I know it's strange to hear this coming from a man, but being a woman is not about prioritizing everyone else over you. It's not about *having* to cook, clean, shop, provide, and make sacrifices all the time.

That's never the way to prove to a man that you are worthy of his love, to kids that you are a good mother, and to a boss that she should promote you or even to yourself that you're doing a good job.

If any part of life feels like a struggle or attracts too much drama to your liking, it's time to realign your role in that part with your strengths, with what your female powers were meant to be used for. Everything costs so much less energy when your life is aligned with who you are.

As I always say in my books, you are the most important person you'll ever meet. You were there from the start and will be present till the very end. You deserve to treat yourself as such. You're a big deal in your own life.

Everyone ought to be true to who they want to be; and if other people then freak out, that's their responsibility, not ours.

Every "yes, sure I'll do it" comes with a price.

The Types of Women Caught Snoozing

Lao Tzu, the ancient Chinese philosopher, once said, "If you are depressed, you are living in the past. If you are anxious, you are living in the future. If you are at peace, you are living in the present."

I'm personally not a huge fan of the "living in the now *all the time*" movement, considering I like to think back on great memories and love to plan for the future. What this chapter is about, however, is seeing something in the now and ignoring it.

When I had just started coaching women, I caught many women snoozing in life, with their eyes wide open. They saw what was going on, but for some reason, they were too sluggish to do anything about it. I've got to admit I was no different in the past. Everyone can sometimes be so indifferent to the real causes of their predicaments that moles have more clarity.

I am sure you have had a friend who found herself in trouble. As she explained what was going on, the solution was clear as day. To you, that is. She, however, seemed unable to acknowledge it.

Think of the woman who continues to spend time on a guy who's clearly never going to change his disrespectful behaviors, but she hangs onto those very few drops of affection he produced in the past. Or the woman who keeps working for a boss who's never going to acknowledge her strengths, while he does *love* to focus on her weaknesses.

All types of women can suffer for a variety of reasons. Yet two categories of women suffer the most.

The Nice Girl

The typical "nice girl" is the best example. She tries to be nice and kind to everyone. She tries to impress the men she meets and seeks the affection of her love interest by pleasing him and adapting to what *he* wants. "How about I make you your favorite dinner with bells on while wearing a lace apron and my sexy high heels?"—for a second date. "How about I reschedule my agenda to fit *your* plans?"—after he's been declining dates for a while because he has "a lot going on at work right now."

Although she dislikes disrespectful behavior as much as everyone else and might even complain about it, she hopes her guy will see the light and change on his own ... someday. Sadly guys like that don't have "someday" on their calendars.

Women are often told through fairy tales that men have a high probability of turning from frogs into princes. I, however, tend to stand by the following theory: you always get the man you have chosen. Meaning: he won't change. Ever. When a woman picks a frog, she ends up with a frog. Disrespectful behavior is like a boomerang. Even when you manage to throw it away, it will come back with vengeance.

The nice girl has a profound intolerance to conflict. Her credo is: "if I try harder, if I show him what a good girl I am, if I show him how much *I* like him, he will like me more." Instead of saying: "Look, you seem to have me confused with a woman who would accept this type of behavior. Oh, you want to see me again? I'll call you tomorrow..." and then she never does.

There's nothing that kills the attraction in a relationship faster than overcompensating and a massive eagerness to please.

The true nice girl will not only feel that something is missing during the dating stage of a relationship, this sense of emptiness continues in later stages too. She'll notice that her husband doesn't treat her the way she deserves to be treated, or at least not the way he used to. She's not getting what she needs from her love life, that's for sure. It's as passionless as the good old phone book. Her guy is often just giving her the minimal amount of investment required to make her stick around. She, on the other hand, puts more and more energy into it, in hopes of turning it around.

And it's not just with her lover that she finds herself in trouble. If the nice girl tries to be a nice mother to her kids, as in the best mother who puts everything aside for the wellbeing of her children (the only definition of mother she knows), she will find herself stuck as well. Some women report feeling they're running on "adrenaline" alone and are balancing on the edge of a cliff. Children also have a tendency to not be very respectful when you try to please *them* all the time.

The same happens at work, where she has a hard time saying no, standing up for herself, and stating her boundaries. And even when she does state them, others cross them with the same ease as they cross any street. Whenever there's a conflict, the nice girl just tries to please harder.

Overcompensating and that massive eagerness to please aren't very compatible with "getting respect" either.

The nice woman's life cannot be anything less than a very emotional roller coaster. She's always at the whim of what she believes other people want from her. Her circumstances define how she feels, and she believes she has no control over it all.

Nice women are not living *their* lives. They might as well be actresses trying to portray the character they feel other people want to see.

I love the nice girl. She has such an open and caring heart, and as soon as she learns to not give in so soon she can become a great high-value woman.

The woman who follows the standard script of life

The pleasing nice girl is, of course, not the only woman who suffers. Women who try to follow the normal script of life—get good grades, get a good job even though you may not like it, work hard until you are old, enjoy the time you have left, the end—eventually get in trouble too.

Oftentimes just trying to juggle taking care of the household, the kids if there are any, the pets, the hubby if there is one, the career—can get them in trouble. From what I hear, hubbies are even harder to raise than kids!

These days, women have to bear that huge weight all on their own. Sure, if they're lucky they find a good guy who tries to help out. He may take out the trash the fourth time she asks. When they travel, he may think of bringing the passports to the airport all on his own, and he may or may not remember their anniversary some years—great guys are out there. They're just a bit harder to find.

But still, it's not the same. When push comes to shove, these women are on their own, and all the responsibilities seem to weigh down upon their shoulders. At least that's what it felt like to a lot of women I've helped over the years.

Furthermore, through no fault of their own, many women seem to live in what I call reaction mode. They react to what happens around them, instead of being in control. Life feels like they're always busy averting some crisis or fixing some problem (often caused by someone else). They're never on their own path.

They might try to be nice in an effort to be liked. They might try to ignore disrespectful behavior from a loved one because they don't want to be a nag. Or, on the contrary, in an effort to not get hurt in the big mean world they might shield themselves off too much from everything that's exciting. They avoid the chaos and the drama, but their life consequently is more boring than gazing at two turtles playing chess.

On top of that, there's a large group of women who give away their power to other people freely. Think of the woman who changes her hobbies because her boyfriend or husband believes they are silly, the woman who worries because her boss said "hello" to everyone this morning but not to her, the woman who gets mad because another person doesn't behave the way he or she should have.

Whenever we react with strong emotions to the outside world and what other people do and don't do, we give them the key to how *we* feel. And without realizing it we just became their servants.

When we get mad, jealous, or feel hurt because of someone else, we allow *them* to make us suffer and feel bad.

It's on us.

That's a mistake. If they don't call us mom or dad, it's not our job to raise other people.

The high-value woman stops people at the gate. She makes sure that she's the one who decides how she feels. She's not perfect by any means. She also feels emotions like anger, jealousy, loneliness, contempt, and anxiety. The difference is she will not act upon them. She understands these are just emotions, a form of energy. Two-year-olds on a sugar rush who are past naptime make better decisions than your emotions do. You should never trust them.

More often than not your emotions are totally wrong and uncalled for if you look objectively at what happened.

Have you ever felt anxiously worried about all that could go wrong during an upcoming event, only to have that actual day pass by peachy, without troubles?

Have you ever felt jealous only to find out, later on, there was no reason to? But you may or may not have acted upon that jealousy first and behaved like a fool. I know I have.

Your emotions alone are never a good guide. They are not oracles; they are mere signs that something *could* be wrong. Emotions are biological signals that try to push us in a certain direction, but it could be the wrong one. You should trust them as much as a little kid standing with a ball in his hand next to a broken vase claiming, "It wasn't me. It fell down on its own." And you should especially never allow other people to control them.

It seems easier said than done. Here's how the high-value woman deals with it. Whenever she feels a strong emotion she takes a step back to distance herself from that emotion. She does so by asking the question: "Why am I feeling this way? What happened?" Then she states, "What's the best way to deal with what just happened, regardless of what my emotions are telling me?"

30

That's it. That's all it takes. I started to practice this over a decade ago, and it became the new automated way my mind reacts to emotions. And if I—part of the emotionally flawed breed of men—can do it, you definitively can!

Long story short, the high-value woman doesn't hit the snooze button and takes control. She does what's best for her in the long run, regardless of how that will make her feel in the short term. She doesn't follow any of society's plans besides her own.

It's Not Your Fault!

If you recognize yourself in what I have been describing, it's important to know that this is not your fault either! I'm not just saying that to make you feel better. Plenty of things that go wrong in your life are the results of your own foolishness. This isn't one of them.

Many studies have shown that women come *programmed* to put the needs of others before their own. A study done in 2014 by Harvard and published in *Harvard Business Review*[6] proves that the reason most men have better careers than the women they married is because married women prioritize their partner's careers above their own. They take a step back to care for the kids and the household—even though they often still work full time—so their man can rise and shine. How kind of them.

It turns out some women act like this in every area of their lives, not just their careers. I have nothing against this phenomenon if it's done with love, respect, and equality within that particular private or work relationship. Most couples are great teams and strengthen one another. But that, of course, isn't always the case.

What's interesting is that this "men first" principle is not part of your primal instincts as a woman. It has been programmed by society. Your primal instincts are all about equality. Mark Dyble, an anthropologist from the University College London, found that our ancestors lived in groups where men and women were

---

[6] https://hbr.org/2014/12/rethink-what-you-know-about-high-achieving-women

indeed equals.[7] Humans are genetically *designed* to be equals and to need each other to survive. So, a woman should never ever accept adapting herself to a man who doesn't do the same nor to a job that doesn't care enough about her needs.

That's what equality is. Both parties adapt, care, and love each other. Even your job should "love" you deeply and allow you to fall sound asleep at night—as if it just told you a bedtime story—instead of keeping you awake. Everyone has a finite amount of time and energy to spend, so be mindful to spend it on things that are energizing and happifying you most of the time.

You deserve to be treated well.

For instance, and this comes as a surprise to some women, *every man* knows how to treat a woman well. When a man likes a woman, he will treat her like a queen. He will protect and take care of her. Chivalry is in his genes.

As I often say in my dating books, when a man claims he loves a woman, but his actions don't show an effort to take care of his queen, to protect her, to help her, to hold her in his arms, consider this a major red flag.

Every guy out there knows how to treat a woman well. So, when a man doesn't, he's doing it on purpose.

Bad men only invest the absolute minimum into the relationship to still get what they want and need. When a man is unwilling to adapt at all to his woman, he may not be into her anymore. Some

---

[7] *Social Structure of Hunter-Gatherer Bands* - M. Dyble et al, *Science* 15 May 2015: Vol. 348, Issue 6236, pp. 796-798 DOI: 10.1126/science.aaa5139

women will then try to conform themselves more in an ultimate effort to rekindle his love. That's a big mistake.

The high-value woman expects her man to adjust just as much as she does. When he doesn't, she won't complain. She starts to ignore him, and she'll focus more on what's important to her (hobbies, passions, career, friends). If he still doesn't turn around, he will say, "Honey, did you change the locks? My key doesn't work ... and are those suitcases in the driveway mine? They look very similar to the ones I've got."

The same goes for a job. I believe everyone should find a job where your unique talents are appreciated. There are companies or clients that will absolutely love you for it. Just as with men, there are a lot of bad companies out there that play you, string you along, and generally don't care about your well-being. They think you're very replaceable. And, of course, to an extent everyone is. But there are professional activities out there that will connect with you on such a level that it's a true win-win. All you need to do is keep looking until you find them.

Finding a great career or job is like dating. You'll meet a lot of frogs before a prince comes along. It personally took me three years to find a company I absolutely *loved* working for. Had I won the lottery, I would have worked there for free. Four years later, the company was sold, and the new owners changed the name into "all profits and no fun." That's when I called it quits and started on my own. These are risky and difficult decisions, but I've learned from studying high-value people that *this* is what they do. They have standards, and they never accept anything that's below their standards for as long as they have a choice. It's only when they don't have a choice that they'll work on accepting and living with it.

Start acting instead of procrastinating.

I can't emphasize this enough. You are great. You are unique. There's nobody— not a single living organism—out there, like you. Nobody looks exactly like you, talks exactly like you, thinks exactly like you ... you are a big deal! You have very interesting gifts to give to the world and great experiences and feelings to get in return. You deserve to come first.

Have Others Pay the Price

As I'm sure you are well aware, you are worth a lot.

We've just established that you are unique, that you are awesome, that the people who get your attention are lucky to be getting it. But the question is, how cheap is your attention, and what price do others have to pay? How much are you selling your attention and affection, your care and love, for?

Here's an excellent formula for instantly being taken for granted: freely give your attention, love, and affection, regardless of how others treat you.

High-value women believe their attention is worth a lot. They love to give and care, but they choose when and who to give it to. As I'll repeat often, they give attention to the people who behave well and ignore the people who don't. This is how they are constantly "training" everyone around them. And since few people like to be ignored, this works remarkably well.

Five years ago, one of my sister's friends had a dating issue. She was recently divorced and had met a great new guy who liked her a lot. That was a fact, given that he had told her so. She had a tendency of taking what men say at face value, so his statement meant the world to her. At least now she was sure of his feelings.

Sadly, his actions were proving otherwise, and she still had to learn you can't take what men say at face value. He had already canceled five dates with a variety of excuses ranging from "I'm held up at work" to "an old friend is in town just for tonight and he wants to meet," and even "Fido, my dog, is a bit sick today. I'm gonna have to cancel." She was mad but disguised it considering she understood all too well that nagging and complaining

36

wouldn't get her far. Unfortunately, she forgot to realize her current behavior wasn't getting her anywhere either.

"He's one of the good guys!" she told my sister and me. "He always made up for it by asking to see me again."

Nonetheless, she had some subtle challenges there too. He often called to ask her out on a same-day date. As in, "Hey, I have time right now. You free?" She always accepted and cleared her schedule. Why wouldn't she? He called and took the initiative. Then there is no problem, right?

Think about it this way. What price was he paying for her attention? What price was he paying to be able to enjoy her company, her affection, her body, her conversation, and her delicious gluten-free lasagna?

Nada, nothing. He kept getting what he wanted regardless of his own behavior and investment. He just had to show up.

"Yeah, I shouldn't do that," she admitted when I called her out on it. "But I love him." Sure, that makes everything all right. It's a trap many fall into.

The high-value woman, on the other hand, always makes others pay a price. Especially when they misbehave like this clown here.

We'll get back to our example in a minute, but let's go over the concept first.

By having others pay a price, they decide how much you are worth to them. That's a pretty strange thing to say, I agree. It was odd to me too, given that I used to discount myself heavily when I was younger, exactly in an effort *to be* liked.

Now if I ask you to think of the people you respect the most, I am willing to bet they are those who clearly show their boundaries. Their attention doesn't come cheap, and when boundaries are crossed, a price has to be paid in the form of an apology or working hard to regain their trust and respect.

Am I right?

This was the case for all of the high-value people I studied, both women and men. That's why they are respected, seen as charismatic, and loved by so many people. When they give attention, you feel important.

That's the true secret of a charismatic person by the way. When you have dinner with a nobody, he will try to convince you he's really important. When you share a meal with a truly charismatic person, he will make *you* feel important. Charismatic people's attention means something and is worth a lot.

Although I'll often use relationship examples because they are easy to identify with, everything I explain in this book extends far beyond romance. This is about *any* form of relationship with another human being, even a stranger you've known for five minutes.

The "for free" price tag my sister's friend was proudly wearing had wreaked some havoc in the past as well, and not just in her romantic relationships. She unsurprisingly had always had bad luck with men. Her husband divorced her and left her for another woman. And at work, she saw others rising faster to the top, even though their performance was not as good as hers. She had a hard time standing out. Whatever group of people she found herself in, for some reason, they always started to wipe their feet off on her, the doormat. And not just in her private relationships! She was the truest version of the nice girl.

The solution was simple. What was she going to be worth from now on? Was she going to be a cheap or high-value woman? She logically chose the latter. Making the transition was tough, but she saw no other choice.

As of that moment, whenever her lover canceled a date, she said, "Sure, have fun! I'll make other plans. Gotta go!" with an enthusiastic voice. No nagging, no complaining. And then she truly disappeared from his radar. She didn't contact him at all, and if he messaged her, it took her days to reply. Not because she was playing games! She simply forced herself to find better things to do.

Guess what happened: *his* behavior changed. He started to put in a much greater effort to see her and to be with her. The next date after she had raised her price, he prepared a fully home-cooked three-course meal, and she got an extensive full body massage for desert, with strawberries and whipped cream *everywhere*. He lavished her with attention like he had never done before.

Men always know how to treat a woman well, even when they seem to have forgotten.

He no longer canceled dates either. She had clearly moved up on his importance ladder. But we weren't there yet. He still called for same-day dates, expecting her to clear her schedule. For some reason, in his mind, his time was more important than hers.

That's when she started to raise her price some more. She said, "No, I can't today. I already have plans," even when all she had to do was alphabetically organize her sock drawer. "We'll hang out another time. Bye!" making him less important. This wasn't a game either. If he showed her behavior like this—thinking she must have nothing else on her mind than waiting for him—her socks truly became more important than him.

Before long, his entire behavior changed. They moved in together about four years ago and are thinking about starting a family. What a transformation! And all she did was raise her price.

Instead of seeking his approval, adapting, and making her attention cheap, she showed him her boundaries. And since he truly cared for her, he gladly accepted and respected them.

We, however, have to show our boundaries to everyone that comes close to us.

Invisible boundaries do not work.

Other people can't guess where they are.

For nearly every woman I have coached, there's often an area in their lives (i.e., professional, romantic, friends, family, children) where they are finding it hard to have others pay a price when boundaries have been crossed.

I've coached successful businesswomen who were real bad-asses in the boardroom that could make pretentious grown-up men cry, but they became approval-seeking doormats at home—and vice versa!

A good rule of thumb here is to listen to your gut. If something doesn't feel right in a certain relationship, for whatever reason, you're probably underpricing your attention and care!

Turn on your self-awareness, and figure out whether you are clearly stating your boundaries to others and whether you have put your foot down or not when the line was crossed. Then make sure you play with your attention. Give attention to the behavior you like (e.g., respecting your boundaries), and ignore the other person when they misbehave. If there is an egregious violation of your boundary, state it clearly and *then* ignore the other person.

There is no better way to get others to respect you more and treat you like they should.

Having others respect your boundaries in *each area* of your life might make some people reject you, but in the long term, this will hurt a lot less compared to when you reject yourself by letting others who are just out to use you, happily walk all over you.

Having Clear Boundaries

To be empowered, stating your boundaries is important, as we've just learned. But there is a right and a wrong way to do so.

As you've read in the previous chapter, other people will never know where your boundaries lie *unless* you show them. You can't assume they are sufficiently intelligent to know what respectful behavior is and isn't or what kind of behavior is or isn't acceptable.

Secret boundaries never work out well. They are the ones that create resentment in the end. You will internally get madder and madder at someone who perpetually crosses your secret boundary, but the question always is: have you pointed out your boundary? "They should know" is never a good answer, especially not when it comes to men.

And as always, what I describe is not just meant for romantic relationships.

I once worked for a company where the founder had no boundaries. He always expected other people to know what he did or didn't like. When an employee did something wrong, he jokingly made some remark that made it perfectly *unc*lear whether he was serious or not. I don't need to explain how bad that was for the company culture. The employees didn't get it indeed. Who could blame them?

If a boundary crossing happens at work by a colleague who gives a totally unnecessary and hurtful remark, you assertively state, "Thank you, that was *really* valuable input" with an accompanied eye-roll and then ignore the other person and continue with whatever you were working on. Or you say, "Thanks, Bob, but if

I need your productive feedback, I'll make sure to come and ask for it."

The good news is most people will not respond like jerks. If they attune themselves to you, they will say something like, "I'm sorry, I shouldn't have said that."

That apology wouldn't have happened if you hadn't stated your boundary first. That's why it's so important.

Although all of this may sound really obvious, you may be someone who tends to stay quiet so you don't hurt the relationship. So let this sink in. If your compliance is the only reason people stay, is it even a relationship at all? If telling the truth or showing your boundaries causes someone else to leave, they'd better pack their bags and leave fast!

I personally love it when I force others to take off their masks. When someone is harsh to me, I say, "Are you having a bad day?" They often take off their angry mask and say, "Yes, I'm sorry. I..."

When I point out a boundary and say, "It's not necessary to talk to me in that way" and they quip back by calling me an idiot, I'm glad too. Now I know for sure I shouldn't invest any more of my time in them. When you state your boundaries, other people don't have to guess how to treat you well. So if they still don't, you'll know it was not an accident.

Who Do You Want to Be?

The most excellent piece of bad advice anyone can ever give you is "Just be yourself!" Maybe you've been on the receiving end of one of these examples:

- "Oh, don't worry. You'll do great during that extremely competitive job interview that can make or break the rest of your career and the lives of generations to come. Just be yourself!"

- "Oh, you're worried about that first date? Don't! Just be yourself. Dating is easy! A walk in the park!"

- "Your wedding vows? Easy! Just be yourself. Who needs to impress anyone anyway? It's not like it's *that* important of a day, is it?!"

Sounds easy indeed, at least to the person handing out the advice.

In the real world where the rest of us live, it just isn't that straightforward. The question remains, who are you? And who do you want to be?

Let's take a deep dive into why it's such an important question in the first place.

If we don't decide who we are, other people and fate will decide it for us! Life will just happen, and we'll be in the back of the bus staring out the window at the road behind us, instead of driving and deciding where to go *and* who to allow on board.

If you just react to your circumstances, to what the men in your life do, to what your colleagues do, to whatever obstacle you face, you won't be in control.

This will be especially important in those circumstances that make you feel emotional. Your emotions are less trustworthy than a foreign undercover spy, as discussed. When you are emotional, it becomes all too easy to respond in the wrong way.

Just ask the already overweight woman who keeps taking *just one more scoop* of ice cream because her emotions tell her she deserves it after such a hard day at work. Or the nice girl who keeps tolerating her cheating and all too often drunk boyfriend because her emotions give her fear when she contemplates breaking up. Or the woman who keeps working long hours for an insatiable boss, when all she wants is to spend more time with her son and to leave at a reasonable hour every day. These people may seem to "just be themselves," but it isn't getting them to where they want. All of these examples are due to not managing emotions with intelligence.

What if making decisions and getting rid of unwanted emotions could become easier? What if you would automatically respond like a high-value woman regardless of the challenges you faced? I'm starting to sound like an infomercial, but it's not as hard as you may think.

Big companies like Apple have mission statements. The entire world knows what they stand for, and customers know exactly what they will and will not get when purchasing one of their products. Moreover, the employees know what the company stands for as well, and this makes it a lot easier for them to make decisions that align to that mission statement. And it's in this easier decision making that lies the secret power of the mission statement.

I noticed that high-value people, although they are not a company, have a personal mission statement too. They decide who they want to be and then find it so much easier to navigate through the obstacles of life because the guidelines have been set *beforehand*.

What's miraculous is that when life throws them a curveball, they're back on their feet a whole lot faster compared to other people who are often still bathing in self-doubt, unsure of what to do. They bounce back faster because they know *where* to bounce back.

Imagine a woman who has this sentence in her personal mission statement: "My health comes first." That's the one big guideline she lives her life by. She comes home after a long day at work and opens her fridge. It's empty. She opens the freezer, it's empty; besides a bucket of ice cream from a party a couple weeks back. Now she could have sworn the ice cream was whispering, "Go ahead. Live a little! Take me, I'm yours any way you want me!"

The decision, however, is easy. Her health comes first. She closes the freezer, knocks on the neighbor's door, and asks if she can borrow some eggs to make herself an omelet.

All of her decisions are made in alignment with her mission statement. There are no doubts; there's no procrastinating. It's easy!

Another woman's mission statement says, "I don't spend time on people who don't respect me."

Now imagine she's in a relationship with a guy who, one year in, decides that it's OK to spend *every* single weekend night with his friends drinking beers instead of doing something fun with her every once in a while. A guy who thinks a romantic date is something you do *before* you're in a relationship, not during. How hard will it be for her to decide if she should dump this fella? It becomes easy. Feeling unhappy about it, hoping that he will change, complaining, or nagging doesn't fit in her personal mission statement. If she has to *ask* for respect, she is, by definition, not respected. Even though her emotions may scream to not do it, she will let him go fast. She knows what she stands for, and she makes decisions accordingly. "Who am I? What do I stand for? What am I about? And is *this* situation compatible with that mission statement?" It's the compass that makes life so much easier.

Kathy, one of my clients, had a tendency of letting others walk all over her. Coming from a past where she had been bullied, she often felt ashamed and had a hard time speaking up. Everywhere! Speaking up, in her mind, was arrogant.

Sitting in a restaurant one day with some colleagues, the waiter brought her plate. She had ordered vegetarian lasagna, but for some reason, the waiter must have heard French fries and a steak since that's what she got.

Old Kathy would have felt some inner resistance. "Do I say something about this? Do I ruin it for everybody? What do I do? I don't want to be a nag." New Kathy, however, had a new mission statement that, all the way at the top, stated: *I come first.*

"Waiter," she said. "This is not what I ordered."

"Sure it is!" the waiter replies. "I remember you ordering a steak medium rare and fries!"

This reaction would have pushed old Kathy off balance. Not so with new Kathy.

"It's really important to me that you take this back to the kitchen and bring me the vegetarian lasagna that I ordered. Can you please do that, John?" now stating the name on his nametag and bringing this sentence with an enthusiastic and authentic smile that communicates: "John, I know you'll do it in the end anyway, so let's save ourselves both the time. Thank you very much!"

And that's exactly what John did. There was no negotiation, no back and forth. Kathy knew the end result she wanted, and that was the only option. John knew that too. The boundary was clear.

This reaction may sound very obvious to you, but it sure wasn't to Kathy. Being a vegetarian, old Kathy would have probably just eaten the fries and the tiny leaf of lettuce.

So how did Kathy, in particular, go about her transformation?

Kathy always admired women who were totally self-sufficient. Women who remained passionate, joyful, and energized regardless of what life was throwing at them. Most of the TV shows and movies she loved featured these types of women and every time she watched her favorite characters in action, she felt energized afterward.

It became clear *that* was who she wanted to be.

So her mission statement was easy: "I'm going to show up with a smile, regardless of what life throws at me. I'll just keep knocking it out of the park. And if it doesn't budge, I'll knock some more. Still with enthusiasm! I'll always bring my best self to every predicament I find myself in. I will no longer let other people dictate how I feel, nor will I accept them walking all over

48

me. I can't control the actions of other people, but I sure *can* mine."

Once her mission statement was in writing, she started to live by it.

Moving forward, the version of herself she described in her mission statement is who she wants to be. Whenever she's in doubt, whenever she's off track, she aligns with her mission statement and continues to follow it diligently no matter how hard it is at first. It serves the most important goal of all— becoming who she is.

At first, this was hard. So I gave Kathy a trick. When in doubt, she simply had to ask herself, "How would my favorite character on TV respond to this?" and that eventually evolved into, "According to my mission statement that defines who I am, how should I respond?"

And now Kathy responds automatically in the way that serves who she really is deep down.

Everything we keep repeating eventually becomes a habit until we no longer have to consciously think about, as plenty of scientific studies have proven.[8] Since we repeat it, the mind concludes it must be important and turns it into an automation. So we'd better think well about what it is we are repeating. Do we have empowering or obstructing habits?

Is this easy?

---

[8] https://www.ncbi.nlm.nih.gov/pmc/articles/PMC3505409/, "the psychology of 'habit-formation' and general practice"

No, far from it! The beginning is hard because most people never take the time to write down their mission statement in the first place. They don't decide who they want to be and keep acting and reacting on autopilot since that's easier in the short term. But you know what? *That* autopilot may have been programmed in the wrong way.

If we don't consciously do this exercise, "who we are" is often just a combination of habits that we've built up in the past. If we've always responded in the bad way, our mind keeps doing it simply because it's a habit. That's why you may see someone encounter the same relationship problems regardless of whom she's dating, or the same professional challenges regardless of where she works.

We need to diligently choose what behaviors we turn into habits. That's why we're going over the most important habits of high-value women all throughout this book.

In order to make life a lot easier, you'll first have to answer the most important question out there. Let's have a look at it in the next chapter.

The Mythical Question

Questions are important. As kids, we have at times been utterly irritating versions of ourselves where everyone we met got attacked by a non-stop barrage of questions going from: "Why do zebras look like horses that couldn't decide what color to wear?" or "Mommy, where do you keep my manners?" to "Mom, I think I'm pregnant, what now?" (Asked by yours truly as a 4-year old boy).

Questions are important because they are stepping-stones to thinking out-of-the-box and seeing something that was previously impossible to view. Had people never asked if the earth was flat, we might never have found out the truth.

Everything humankind now takes for granted in the world was seemingly impossible at one point in time until someone asked the right questions.

Think about it. The fact that everyone uses *wireless* devices and is able to talk to other people and surf the web using a device as tiny as a pack of dollar bills is amazing. "Impossible!" would have been the response had you tried to explain it to someone in the 1930s. Yet, the technology has *always* been there. We didn't get a cargo drop from an alien spaceship with new technology or materials that weren't already present on Earth. Everything was here, but nobody had asked the question yet.

Martin Cooper, the inventor of the cell phone, did ask himself the question: "What if I could make a phone call from wherever I am, wherever I stand, without needing a wire?" That question led him to invent the first wireless phone in the seventies.

If we want to change the problems we have, the way people respond to us, the successes we have and miss out on, or even how happy we feel, we need to ask better and different questions.

And it all begins with the mother of all questions: "Who do I want to be?"

The answer always appears at the very top of our mission statement.

That's quite a mythical question, isn't it? It's one very few people take the time to answer. Whether you're aiming for a 1 percent change or a massive transformation, you need to ask questions.

Let's make it easier by slowly building up to the master question.

What areas in your life do you feel resistance in? What parts seem to attract drama? These will be the parts of your life where you are off track and not aligned with your *true* self. Your habitual responses there may not be serving you.

How are you currently responding to the events in *that* area of your life (e.g., I often feel anxious, frustrated, jealous, sad, mad, lonely, lazy, or helpless)?

How would the ideal version of you respond in those specific situations?

Which amazing women do you absolutely love? How are they responding to difficult circumstances? What is it about their personalities that you would love to transplant into yours? Is it their passion? Their positive outlook? Their confidence? The fact that they seem to love life no matter what? That they always bring their best selves? What is it? What is it they stand for? What is important to them?

What do other people you admire stand for? What may be in their mission statement?

What would *you* like to stand for?

What do you want to be known for?

Try to get into the details, and come up with answers like:

- "I want to stand up for myself and clearly show my boundaries, even when I'm afraid."
- "I want to be kind and never bitter."
- "I still care about others and will help where I can, but I put myself first."
- "I no longer run away from making difficult decisions. I won't fear making a bad one. I will make the decision that aligns with my mission statement and see where it brings me."
- "I will bring passion to everything I do."
- "I value loyalty more than anything else. I will always be loyal, but will only keep giving attention to those who are loyal to me."
- "I value friendship above everything else."
- "I value health above everything else."
- "When I feel I'm not in line with who I am, I will correct my course no matter what scares me."
- "I will not get mad at myself when I've made a bad decision. I'd rather make a bad decision than be indecisive."
- "I will never change my actions in an effort to be liked."
- "I put myself first, so in the end, I have more to give to others."
- "I will screw up, and that's totally fine!"

- "I no longer bottle up my emotions. I will kindly share my feelings when someone has overstepped a boundary, regardless of the consequences."
- "I'd rather be single than be in a relationship that doesn't make me happy."
- "I'd rather have people reject me than have them walk over me."

These are just some examples that can go into your mission statement, and yours can, of course, be totally different. As soon as you get the answers, you'll have inserted the right destination into your navigation system of life, and when you find yourself procrastinating about anything, it will be a lot easier to see what the right course of action is.

Can you imagine how much this simplifies life?

Imagine a woman named Karen who has in her mission statement: "For me, family always comes first."

Tonight, her sister is going to perform on stage at her first mini-concert, and she asked her to come and watch. Karen, a hard-working woman, is about to leave work when her boss swings by and says, "We will need you to stay late tonight. There's an important problem we would like you to take a look at...."

Had Karen not taken the time to write down her mission statement she might have wondered what to do. She had promised her sister, but if she doesn't stay late now, she may lose her job....

This will be a tremendously difficult decision to make. Whatever she chooses, it will be a lose-lose situation. If she stays, she's going to feel bad for her sister. If she goes, she's going to be afraid she upset her boss. She won't feel well either way.

With her mission statement in mind, however, the decision becomes much easier. After a quick consideration and weighing the outcome, she says in a friendly way: "I'm really sorry. I can't tonight. I'm happy to stay late on another day like I have before, but I already have plans tonight. I'm going to see my sister perform on stage, and it's important both to me and her. I can't cancel it." And that's that. Karen is very flexible otherwise and has changed plans before; this time, however, she can't.

Even though she wants to help out when she can, she knows that if she is not aligned with who she *really* is, the daily frustration she will feel will be a lot worse than the guilt she may feel tonight. She can always work late on another day—and she does so often—but she can never recover the family moment she will miss out upon on this particular night.

She has thought well about her mission statement. *Family first.*

Needless to say, for some people it will be "my career first." I'm not here to suggest what's best since, as discussed, this mission statement is unique to everyone.

Life becomes so much easier, and making decisions is automated when you have thought out your mission statement. Many perpetual loops of worry will vanish and won't reappear.

And let's be honest, if Karen delivers good work otherwise, her saying no will have no consequences whatsoever. Others, her boss included, will often respect her *more* because she respectfully stands up for herself.

It's never, ever your responsibility to give other people everything they wish for from you anyway!

That's a game you cannot win. They will keep wishing until there's nothing left.

For at least one week, decide that you will react and act as if you are that better version of yourself. Consider the sentences you write down during this exercise your roadmap. Just give it a try for seven to fourteen days to see what it feels like. I bet you won't want to return to the old way of thinking.

You can do the mission statement exercise now or when you're done reading the entire book, but please start asking the right questions to arrive at your mission statement. The impact on your life will be so big that you may wonder why they don't teach this in schools.

Now the next time someone tells you to just be yourself, you will know who that is!

When It Hurts, Get the Band-Aids

Wouldn't it be great if life were perfect? Like happily ever after perfect? What if you could enjoy every day without *having* to worry about anything? A life where absolutely nothing was going wrong.

Isn't that what you should all work toward?

That mythical life seems to exist since it's advertised so often and portrayed by real human beings on social media and sorts. Yet, it's nothing but a hoax. You have a better chance of succeeding in teaching a rabbit French than ever living a life free of obstacles and problems. Obstacles are everywhere, for everyone.

The problem with normal obstacles is they don't hurt tremendously. We think we can safely put it off and deal with it later. It's something that "future us" can handle. Postponing is totally fine for some challenges but not for many.

If you accidentally cut your finger, how long would it take you to get the disinfectant and some Band-Aids? How long before you took action?

You would do it right away, of course. Waiting would be silly because the wound could get infected, you might get a fever, and eventually die and leave everyone wondering why you decided to forgo the trip to the medicine cabinet. You probably never thought of it that way and I realize I'm over-dramatizing, but you still go get the disinfectant and take care of the problem.

But why?

Is there a huge problem now? It's just a small cut and some blood

... yet, you instinctively know that if you don't take care of it *right now*, problems may follow. It's just the right thing to do.

When it hurts and bleeds, you get the Band-Aids because you instinctively think of the long-term consequences of not acting right away.

Nevertheless, for other obstacles, you may decide to waste time (since there is no blood) and be lazy. You will act when you're absolutely forced to. I'm not pointing fingers here, besides the one at myself. I've been found waiting for obstacles to clear up on their own more than once in the past. There was no blood, but it did cost me dearly on some occasions.

When there is an obstacle in your path, it's better to not look away and deal with it. Remove it, dig a tunnel under it, make your way next to it. Don't wait. It's costing you time, money, love, and fun.

The high-value woman always keeps the long term in mind, her ultimate destination, *and* she makes sure she's passionate about the journey while getting there. She has trained herself to love dealing with obstacles. She understands they come with life and even then she chooses to bring her best self each and every time.

Having a great life is a constant work-in-progress. Problems are a given, for everyone, and I found that the people who learned to enjoy solving their problems are the happiest.

Marcia came to see me a couple of years ago. She had been waiting for her obstacles to disappear on their own for such a long time that she had finally had enough of it. Marcia was seriously overweight, had bags under her eyes, and frizzled hair. She looked unhealthy and told me she was tired all the time. It was pretty clear why: she couldn't stop eating sugary desserts, and she was drinking three macchiatos every day and two to three glasses of wine at night to counter the caffeine that kept her up otherwise. Before bed, she ate a bag of chips. She told me she longed for it and couldn't resist. After a hard day, she *deserved* all of it. And her days were hard indeed; she experienced roadblocks everywhere and felt stuck.

If we were shortsighted, we might conclude: well, that's clearly who Marcia *is*! She has a longing for it. Her lioness wants to be fed sugar, macchiatos, and alcohol. So for Marcia to align with who she really is, she needs to not feel guilty and eat some more! You go, girl!

That is not how it works, of course.

Truth be told, Marcia felt sick because of who she had become. She showed me pictures of what she looked like ten years ago and the difference was night and day. *This* version of her was clearly not who she was!

Can you already see what's going on with Marcia? Was the barista who always got her name right at fault for all of the macchiatos she drank? Were the sinful cookies even the Pope couldn't resist to blame? Or was something else the real culprit?

She used eating as a way to fill the emptiness inside, but it wasn't her stomach that was feeling empty. Marcia's talents were being ignored at work, she couldn't seem to find a great guy, and jumped from relationship to relationship with men who all started to withdraw after only a couple of weeks or months. And on top of all that, she felt lonely and didn't have any real friends. So to comfort herself, she ate and never stopped.

Marcia was ignoring her power and was camping out in front of her roadblocks. She believed she could not change her predicament and that she was doomed to live this unfulfilling life. And if that's what Marcia really believed, why wouldn't she indulge in everything that she can stomach? What's the point in being healthy anyway?

Obstacles, however, need to be dealt with. And the more we love the process, the better our life will be.

My primary job was to make her see what was really going on: her self-limiting belief was wrong. She had much more power over her predicament than she believed. After that, I had to give her the tools to get out of her mess.

Marcia needed to find projects and passions that could fulfill her body *and* her starved soul. One of the questions I asked Marcia was what she loved doing as a kid, a teenager, and a young adult. Were there any times in life where she was naturally energized, in the flow, and really loving what she was participating in?

She told me she loved to dance and was really good at it. So good that she could have become a pro, but her parents thought she needed a *real* job. Plus, she loved to write short stories. Two totally different passions that equally fulfilled her as a young girl.

I explained to Marcia that eating all that junk could never satisfy her *real* needs. They would remain unmet and would incessantly make her miserable.

Since she had so many self-limiting beliefs, I asked her to try a new strategy for thirty days. Just thirty days. That didn't seem insurmountable to her.

First, I asked her to dance in front of the mirror at home, with a big smile, *even* when she didn't feel like it. Especially then! She could dance any way she wanted. The second assignment was to start writing again, join a book club, or follow a writer's course.

That's it.

I didn't ask her to eat less! She thought that was odd since every coach or therapist she had tried out before *did* focus on her meals and snacks.

Her binge eating was merely a symptom of a deeper problem. If I had asked her to eat less, she might have managed for a little while and then she would have rebounded, considering the causes were still present. You should never spend your willpower—a limited resource—on the symptoms of your challenges. The *causes* are what you need to tackle. Those are the real obstacles.

Please take a moment to let that sink in. Her tiredness and her sugar addiction were not the obstacles! They were merely symptoms of the real obstacle: her starving soul.

So Marcia got started, and sixty days later, she had already lost twelve pounds, the bags under her eyes were almost gone, and her face looked more radiant. She had that attractive glow back.

Long story short, the dancing brought her in touch with her power. It unlocked some of the joy she hadn't felt for years and made her feel empowered. She then used that power to effortlessly say "no" to that cheesecake in her fridge and to everything else that tried to seduce her.

The writing helped her feel like she was creating something meaningful. She now had a purpose that aligned with what had fulfilled her in the past. And the book club and writing course helped her meet like-minded people who became her positive support network, her own mini community.

In sixty days!

She recently sent me an email—it's been seven years since Marcia began her journey—and she now earns a living writing fiction books. She moved to another state where she met her now husband at a writers' conference. She lost more weight, feels energized, and eats healthy. She doesn't even *have* cheesecakes in the fridge anymore.

She made one simple decision. She told herself, "This is who I want to be" and then she became it by dealing with the roadblocks that were standing in her way.

Whenever you meet a roadblock, you need to deal with it just as you would deal with a wound. Don't go camping in front of the important obstacles in hopes of it disappearing on its own.

For so many people, the bad relationship, job, friendships, or health are merely symptoms, not the cause. And yet you may think it is.

You may be tempted to think:
- "Oh, she's unhappy because Bill, her husband, treats her badly."
- "Oh, she's unhappy because she's not being valued at work."
- "Oh, she's unhappy because she's not working on anything meaningful."

These are not the causes! The question is: why does she think she should stay trapped in those situations? Why is she accepting such behavior from others? Why does she sulk and wait for the obstacles to vanish on their own?

We often have much more power over our external problems than we think.

You deserve to have your primary needs met.

That's why I asked you to think about your mission statement, who you want to be, what gives and what costs you energy. That information will help you make decisions and will assist in stopping any procrastination.

Finding a new route when a roadblock pops up is easy when you have a destination in mind.

"Is this compatible with who I am?" is all you'll have to answer to end procrastination and behave like a high-value woman. Since, if the answer is "no," it's time for a change in direction, regardless of what your emotions may be communicating.

And when you're on the right track, you will automatically be tapping into your power. And you'll *have* so much more energy because you won't be spending willpower on the wrong people, the wrong worries, and the wrong tasks.

If you've never practiced this before, you're in for a positive surprise!

But first, let's deal with feeling overwhelmed. When facing many roadblocks at once, it's easy to feel anxious.

How to End Feeling Overwhelmed

With all of the tasks, to-do lists, and responsibilities you have as a woman, it's easy to become overwhelmed.

Stress makes people jittery; anxiety makes them run for the hills. Feeling overwhelmed, however, makes them give up. It stops everything in its tracks.

In the last twenty years, humankind has been feeling bewildered more than ever by the abundance of choices available in life. Eighty years ago, as a woman, you had about six *mandatory* daily decisions:

1. What am I going to cook for breakfast? Eggs? Bacon? Or bacon *and* eggs to make it super fancy.
2. Is it a good idea to hang out the clothes to dry now? Because those clouds don't look very promising.
3. What am I going to cook for lunch? Some pork, corn, and beans?
4. Will I go to the local market for some veggies, or will I pick something from the garden?
5. What am I going to cook for dinner? Some leftover pork, beans, and the tomatoes I picked from the garden?
6. What time should I leave to pick up little Steven from school?

That was about it. All of the other choices could probably wait till morning. And those you had to make weren't all that tough anyway. Few choices could end up in disasters, and you didn't have the constant feeling that you were missing out.

Choices women did not *have* to make those days were: "Should I ask for a raise? What will we eat tonight? I heard there's a substance in beans called lectin that causes a permeable gut wall. So that might be bad. What kind of strange-sounding cup of coffee will I order today, and should I give my real name? They always get it wrong. Where will our next vacation be? Do I pick a hotel, or do I go for a vacation rental? Right, I must not forget to ask for some time off first. Um, I see he read my message, but why isn't he replying? His status says he's online. Should I text him something else, a question maybe? *Do* I want to watch the next episode my TV is proposing? I wonder why cats are so afraid of cucumbers. Should I look that up?"

And this is probably just your average woman's thoughts in a 90-second timeframe.

As a woman, you have the mental capacity to worry at a much higher rate than a man as a result of a difference in neural brain connections, as studies show.[9]

But the problem with all of those options and seemingly important choices is that few women actually make choices!

The solution to ending the sense of overwhelm is to make choices and be done with them.

But what if you make the wrong decision? That's the million-dollar question. There are people who don't decide because they are afraid of making the wrong decision and setting in motion the end of life as they know it. I used to be one of them. I got a spontaneous rash when I even got close to making *any* important decision.

---

[9] Sex differences in the structural connectome of the human brain, M.I., T.D.S., H.H., R.E.G., R.C.G., and R.V.
http://www.pnas.org/content/111/2/823.abstract

Then I learned everyone has regrets. There's nobody walking around on this planet without any regrets. It's impossible not to make bad decisions! You're not clairvoyant, you can't look into the future, so whether you decide or not ... *not deciding* might turn out to be the bad decision.

Make no mistake, "not deciding" is a decision too!

My personal history started to make this blatantly obvious. I was stuck in many areas of my life *because* of my indecisiveness. Not having decided turned out to be the worst decision for many of the proverbial crossroads I still found myself standing at.

Then, when I started to study high-value people, I learned they are really good at deciding. They never procrastinate for long, and they keep moving.

Decide, and if it turns out to be a bad decision, realign your course. Good stuff comes from deciding. Every successful person has had to make a ton of decisions with both good and bad results. It's an inevitable part of life.

One of the most recurring regrets of people on their deathbeds is a certain risk they didn't take but wished they had. They prefer knowing it was the bad decision over not knowing whether it would have been the right one.

Try to get comfortable with making decisions, and make indecisiveness uncomfortable.

High-value women constantly make choices. They are in the driver's seat, not in the passenger seat. And as a driver, you continuously make choices, "What route should I pick? Should I brake for this pigeon or is it just stubbornly pretending it didn't see me? What do I do with that idiot behind me who seems convinced he owns the road and everyone on it?"

Kelly was forty-three when it hit her one morning, like an overdue slap in the face: "What the hell am I doing? I just made breakfast for the kids, then I've got to go to work where I'll look at my computer screen for nine hours only to return home, cook dinner, watch some TV, go to bed, and then it starts all over again. Is this what my life will look like until I'm eighty-four and ready to go to a nursing home?"

It was shortly after this realization that Kelly contacted me. Kelly had married her high school sweetheart, started building a family, and took a job that would allow her to be a good mother. She had set aside most of her dreams (besides starting a family). Then at thirty-four, she and her husband divorced. At forty-three, her kids were seventeen and twenty. She was *still* making them breakfast and taking care of virtually everything she could. "That's what good mothers do," she thought. Kelly didn't have a loving mother herself, and she tried to avoid becoming like *her* at all costs.

That cost was very high indeed.

Having kids and starting a family was one of her dreams, and she achieved it. I've met many women over the years who have dedicated their lives to their lovers and children, and there's nothing wrong with that *unless* they keep sensing that they are missing out on something big. Not on partying and sipping mojitos all night but something much deeper.

Kelly had gotten stuck in a loop that had been going on for about twenty years. She had to take care of so many things that she forgot to take care of herself. Not only had she gained thirty-two pounds over the years, she felt tired and mentally empty all the time, regardless of what kind of vitamins she popped. She was running on empty.

The interesting thing is that Kelly knew all too well what she had to do, but she had been perpetually postponing the decision.

So Kelly finally decided to make a monstrous change: she asked her kids to help in the household. That's it! What a concept. She taught them how to cook and wash as in: "This is how you turn on the dishwasher, this is how you empty it. When you wash clothes, don't put red and white together unless you love pink...." And you know what? They got it! To her surprise, they were smart enough to operate this type of heavy machinery and still get out unharmed.

With all of that time freed up, she started working out and went to a yoga class where she practiced strange poses that made absolutely no sense to her. In that class, however, she met three other women with whom she really connected. Kelly made a pact with them that they were going to visit three new countries every year, on their own. No husbands, boyfriends, or children allowed.

On top of that, she talked to her boss and asked for more meaningful projects to work on. He told her he was glad she finally asked.

These are the only changes she made ... yet in less than twelve months, she looked and felt like a totally different woman. She finally felt alive.

I mention Kelly because she is another prime example of how big an impact small changes can make. She didn't make any earth-shattering shifts. They were subtle (even though they were very difficult to make to her; she felt really guilty asking the kids for help). Yet, they had a huge impact. Kelly had used her power to make decisions that aligned her with who she really wanted to be. That's the woman she finally became.

Before the next chapter, I want to briefly mention Eva. Growing up, Eva had always loved dancing, as do many girls. She spent countless hours dancing in front of the mirror as a child and a teenager. She even took dance lessons and became really good at it. But then, as always, life started to get in the way. She couldn't combine it with her studies at the university. Then she met her husband and before you know it, Eva was forty-seven and hadn't danced in over twenty-seven years.

Eva found me as she was heading toward a burnout at the rate of a speeding bullet.

Instead of suggesting her to work less or to rest, I asked her these questions:

1. When was the last time you were truly full of energy?
2. When was the last time that the clock had stopped ticking, that everything felt exactly right?

After a little insisting from my side, Eva decided to pick up dancing again. At first, it felt strange, because doubt about her age popped up. Her husband didn't help either when he said, "Dancing? At our age?"

Some men—always prime examples of true empathy.

Eva persisted, and even though she had a demanding career, she found time to dance at least three times per week for one hour or more. She also took private dance classes in a dance studio once a week where she perfected her moves. These dance classes had no goal; they weren't meant to achieve anything or win medals, and the dancing was the only change she made in her life. Eva didn't kick her husband to the curb because she loved him and he was one of the good guys. She didn't change her job because she liked the projects she worked on. She didn't go on a diet. She simply made one tiny change.

Eva recently told me that everything else had changed with it. She is happy, more resistant to stress, feels sexier, has more confidence, sleeps better, started working out—and the list goes on and on. All of this because of one little change, one little talent or treasure she had discovered as a teenager and had forgotten all about. All she had to do was make the decision. That was the hardest part. It always is.

To tap into your power, you can make big changes like single-handedly ending world hunger, or you can make tiny changes like the examples we've just explored. The choice is up to you, but I suggest you start with tiny ones to avoid feeling overwhelmed. Then build from there. When it feels right, you're on the right track. Sometimes one tiny change is all that's needed. But whatever you do, don't stop deciding.

The most excellent formula for feeling overwhelmed is to keep procrastinating and pushing aside as many decisions as you can. Don't let the decision balls pile up, just keep knocking them out of the park.

Stop Taking Care of Everything!

As seen in the examples I have shared, the biggest roadblocks that pop up for most women are: I have no time, and I just need to take care of everything and everyone else *first*.

Not really. Nobody says you need to be on call like a flight attendant or be an organizational mastermind like a flight controller.

Now if you suffer from this, you are not alone. You often sense a lack of time exactly because you may have a hard time letting others help out. You may think, "At least then it's done right."

Here's another question: has it ever occurred to you that, especially when there are kids, women seem to take care of *everything* in the household?

Not that they "do" everything. Good men help out a lot. But in many households, it's the woman who's at the reins of the *organization* of it all.

Even though women's brains are better wired to take care of the whole enchilada than men's, that doesn't mean they should!

It's often the willingness of a woman to take care of *everything* that relieves others from having to. Don't give them that freedom. Let them work a bit as well. Everything that you take care of is already marked as *complete* for all of those close to you.

This may be very obvious to you, but if you suffer from overwhelm or too much stress, have a look of what you could stop doing so others can take care of it for you. You're often better off with them helping out and failing here and there (meaning not doing it as well as you would have), than ending in burnout with feelings of exhaustion. Then *everything* fumbles.

Why Feminine Women Get Great Relationships with Masculine Men

I have already mentioned the two types of energy: masculine energy and feminine energy. Masculine energy is about ambition, strength, power, go-getting and crushing it (often literally). Feminine energy is about empathy, (talking about) feelings, emotions, friendship, companionship, and community. Both men and women possess these two forms of energy, meaning that go-getting is not exclusive to men. It's just part of "masculine energy" that women possess as well. Likewise, men can love flowers and companionship, but on average these things will be *more* important to women than they are to men. The fact that there are two energies originates from Yoga philosophy, where male energy is known as Shiva and female energy as Shakti. Ancient Egypt and Greece philosophy also made a clear distinction between masculine and feminine energy. [10] But as scientific studies show, these energies can mostly be seen in the actual differences of behavior between men and women.[11]

---

[10] *The Kybalion – A Study of the Hermetic Philosophy of Ancient Egypt and Greece,* published by Global Grey; Marianne van den Wijngaard (1997). *Reinventing the sexes: the biomedical construction of femininity and masculinity. Race, gender, and science*; Worell, Judith, *Encyclopedia of women and gender: sex similarities and differences and the impact of society on gender,* Volume 1 Elsevier, 2001; Thomas, R. Murray (2000). *Recent Theories of Human Development.* Sage Publications ; Bosson, Jennifer K.; Vandello, Joseph A. (April 2011). "Precarious manhood and its links to action and aggression"; Winegard, Bo M.; Winegard, Ben; Geary, David C. (March 2014). "Eastwood's brawn and Einstein's brain: an evolutionary account of dominance, prestige, and precarious manhood". *Review of General Psychology.* PsycNET; Bassi, Karen (January 2001). "Acting like men: gender, drama, and nostalgia in Ancient Greece". *Classical Philology.* Chicago Journals.

[11] Servin A1, Nordenström A, Larsson A, Bohlin G. Prenatal androgens and gender-typed behavior: a study of girls with mild and severe forms of

Over the more than a decade of coaching men and women in their relationships, I noticed something interesting. First, some men are far from saints. As a man myself, this came as a total shock. The second realization was opposites attract. That was less of a shocker, but it's not in the way most people understand that principle. It has nothing to do with individual tastes or values as in: he loves classical music and wears a bow tie to work, and she listens to death metal and has a middle finger tattooed on her forehead, they must be a great match since opposites attract. It's all and *only* about the energies and never about the values (these should ideally not be opposites).

Masculine energy is attracted to feminine energy and vice-versa. Even same-sex couples will very often have a "man" and a "woman" in that relationship, as you may have noticed.
But that was *still* not the interesting part I discovered.

Soft, feminine women often end up with really masculine men.
Soft, feminine men often end up with really masculine women.

If those soft, feminine women are not high-value women who clearly define their boundaries, they become the doormats of the men they are with. The speed of that process depends on the badness of the man they chose to love. The narcissist will be

---

congenital adrenal hyperplasia.
https://www.ncbi.nlm.nih.gov/pubmed/12760514, D. Bruce Carter1, Laura A. McCloskey Peers and the Maintenance of Sex-Typed Behavior: The Development of Children's Conceptions of Cross-Gender Behavior in Their Peers http://guilfordjournals.com/doi/abs/10.1521/soco.1984.2.4.294, Abbie E. Goldberg, Associate Professor, Deborah A. Kashy, Professor, and JuilAnna Z. Smith Gender-Typed Play Behavior in Early Childhood https://www.ncbi.nlm.nih.gov/pmc/articles/PMC3572788/, Gender Roles and Gender Differences
http://highered.mheducation.com/sites/0072820144/student_view0/chapter15/index.html

dominating her faster than you can say eggplant, whereas the normal bad men will take a bit longer.

The same goes for the soft, feminine man who ends up in a relationship with a strong, masculine woman. She will have bulldozed him over faster than it takes that guy to peel off his daily facemask.

I saw a lot of casualties in the war of love.

Interestingly, *if* that feminine woman *is* in touch with her feminine energy, if she becomes a high-value woman, she can have a fantastic relationship with really masculine men and feel awesome. Mind you, I'm not describing macho men with long beards who run around with axes, pretending to be Vikings. It's still the energy I'm focusing on.

A real high-value masculine man will take care of his woman, even though she can take care of herself. He will be purposeful and have a clear direction of where he wants his life to go.

Here's the kicker: *a real high-value masculine man will not be dazzled when you behave like a woman!*

Please take a moment to let that sink in. Such men will never hold the fact that you are a woman and behave like one against you. On the contrary, it's what attracts them. And most importantly, he will fulfill his woman's deepest desires—outside of the bedroom too. That's what *real* men do!

Too many women never get to experience this, because they either act like men or are afraid to be feminine and shield themselves off. They are afraid to get hurt. I don't blame them. Some may have heard previous boyfriends or husbands complain:

- "Stop being so sensitive!"
- "Why do you always have to make a big deal out of *everything*?"
- "What? A headache? AGAIN?"

These are mumblings coming from men who don't *get* women.

Some women think they want a sensitive and sweet guy, one who's ready to talk about feelings. A BFF so to speak. Someone who knows that it's not just about what you say but also *how* you say it. And even though being with such a sensitive man may sound great in theory, as soon as they get one of these sweet men, they get bored and feel like they're in a relationship with a sensitive brother instead of a lover.

The true magic happens when a woman gets in touch with her full femininity. That's what makes the high-value woman so special and attractive. Even deep into her long-term marriage or relationship, there's still passion because she remains at the peak of her femininity while allowing her lover to be bathing in his masculine energy. She doesn't fear it; she loves it.

If deep down you are a very feminine woman (meaning you are caring, loving, full of empathy, sensitive, don't like hurting anyone), but you decide to hide it, you will continuously attract the wrong type of men. That's why women wonder, "How come the men I'm interested in don't notice me, yet I always attract men I'm not interested in at all?" It's because of that mismatch of energies. You need to show and exude your dominant feminine energy. If you *are* in a relationship and you hide it, you will get very inconsistent behavior from the man you are with. We will dive more into that in a later chapter when I talk about emasculating men.

76

In general, if you build walls around your heart, the right prince can't see his princess.

The Ugly Duckling

Have you ever heard the story of the ugly duckling? It's a story with an important life lesson embedded in it.

As soon as it's born, it doesn't look at all like the other ducklings. Before long, it's pushed out of the nest by mother duck who herself has been pressured by her peers to exile the ugly duckling.

On the run, the ugly duckling is not accepted by anybody. He's laughed at and ridiculed. He doesn't know who he is or where he belongs.

On his search for meaning and love, he encounters other animals that laugh at him too. At some point, he is accepted into the home of an older woman who has a cat and a hen.

They too ridicule the ugly duckling. The cat asks, "What good are you if you can't catch any mice?" and the hen follows up with, "What good are you when you can't lay any eggs?"

The ugly duckling tries to explain he loves to stick his neck underwater to dive and that he loves to fly. The cat cannot understand why anyone would love to swim, let alone *underwater*. The hen, on the other hand, doesn't comprehend why flying could be of any use; *she* never does it.

So the duckling has to leave there too.

Time and time again, the ugly duckling is exiled and scared away. Then one day our ugly duckling is floating on a lake. All of a sudden, he sees two beautiful swans swimming in the distance. The duckling thinks they are the most beautiful creatures he's ever seen.

The swans notice him and start to swim closer. The ugly duckling fears their rejection, since to be rejected by such beautiful creatures would be the worst that could happen to him. He is so afraid that he bows his head.

And there, in the reflection of the water, he sees an elegant swan. He is surprised and not sure what he sees. Seconds later, he realizes he is looking at himself. He *is* a beautiful swan.

He is immediately greeted and fully accepted by the oncoming swans, and they all live happily ever after.

Sometimes, real rejection is good. It forces us to keep looking until we find where we belong. This applies to romantic relationships, where a rejection or loss of interest means it's time for the next one. You'll also find this in your career, where a rejection is a clear sign you belong somewhere else where your unique talents will be more appreciated.

The duckling could have chosen to live with the cat and the hen while never being fully accepted. But he kept looking until it felt right.

You should never try to keep someone or something that doesn't want to keep you.

As obvious as this may sound, it amazes me every single day how many people settle for less, trying to regain the interest of someone who separated from them or trying to keep a job that hasn't pleased them in a very long time. It's a bit masochistic when you think about it.

As the duckling proves, there is something that fits us out there.

If it feels like it doesn't fit right, it's always a good idea to keep on trying new things.

The story of the duckling also relates to the fact that everybody judges. The cat judges and cannot even begin to understand why *anyone* would love water. How could she? It's not *her* thing. That's her judgment. It's just an opinion. We shouldn't try to change it! We cannot get the cat to *like* water. We cannot get some people to understand why we like what we like or why we're different compared to them.

My own mother never understood why I am who I am. She wanted me to be an extrovert, while I'm an introvert. She wanted me to this and that—so I could fit her image of what a good son would be. At first, I tried to comply in an effort to please her. I wanted to take her overall frustrations and pains away, but in the process, *I* was the one who suffered. That's when I decided it's *her job* to deal with it. If she cannot come to terms with how I want to live my life, then it's not up to me to remove her pain and frustration. That is her job. The same goes for everyone else who believes they should mold you into someone different.

Just imagine if the swan had tried to catch mice or stopped flying—just to fit in. Would he be living a great life? One that felt fulfilling? Of course not! Yet, so many people do just that in order to avoid rejection. The pain of rejection is hard, but not living a life that is true hurts significantly more and lasts until you adjust to what your internal navigation system has been saying all along. From now on, learn to welcome rejection. It is a necessary part of life. Every rejection brings you closer to what you really need!

It takes the swan a long time and even a chance of luck to see his real reflection. To see himself for who he really is. So many women and men keep living in that state of denial. They don't even know what a beautiful swan they are because they have been ridiculed in the past or because they haven't found their thing yet. They feel they need to hide themselves because of the reactions they have received from people whose judgments don't matter.

The good news is that it's never lost. The ugly duckling does find out he is a swan after all. It just takes him some additional trial-and-error and perseverance during the challenging times. That's OK. If the story would have continued, I'm sure he would have become a stronger swan than all of the other swans with a safer upbringing. That is usually how it goes in real life as well.

Ice-Cold Women

About sixteen years ago, I had my first real work experience after getting my masters degree. I walked into the big ad agency that decided to hire me and was introduced to my direct boss and mentor: the ice-cold woman. It was my first real encounter with one, and to be honest, I was a bit shaken up about it.

She was around forty, thin, blonde, and pretty. But her eyes— they were so cold, angry, and stressed it actually frightened me. Other people weren't fond of her and were clearly afraid to even enter her office, the very office my desk was located in as well. The words "shark tank" took on an entirely new meaning to me because upon entering her office, you could get devoured in seconds. Not unsurprisingly, men were not attracted to her. Her love life was nonexistent. Even though she looked like a woman and was pretty, she oozed masculine energy that was repelling men.

My career at that firm didn't look very promising the first couple of days since she was my direct boss. But four days in, I saw it for the first time. Karen, the fake name I'm going to use for her, was wearing a mask. Her mask and carefully played-out persona were almost perfect. Yet I happen to be a highly sensitive person, which means that subtle details can catch my attention easily. So the little cracks in her mask, in her acting, became more and more clear as time passed.

Even though she looked like the sternest woman in the entire office, even though she often behaved like a nasty woman, she happened to be the sweetest, most fragile, most hurt woman I have ever met. Ever.

But you wouldn't have seen it by observing her or experiencing her presence. And I'm sure only a few people had seen it or even cared.

But I did and not just because I had to work with her. I have a thing for deciphering enigmas like these. So I brought my hands to her face as slowly as I could, in an effort not to spook her. And I removed her mask bit-by-bit, layer-by-layer until I finally got to see the real Karen.

Honestly, Karen was in deep trouble. As I said, she was a very soft, sensitive, and sweet woman who needed some love, some warmth, some caring and caressing. But nobody, absolutely nobody was giving it to her. Would you, if the person you're interacting with is acting like a bitch? And I don't use that word without reason. Angry rattlesnakes were easier to handle.

What she needed the most: some loving, some attention, some being part of the team were never hers to have because of the stupid mask she chose to wear, day in and day out like a favorite sweater.

The more you wear masks in life, the less other people can see the real you. The less they can see the real you, the worse those very people and the world, in general, are going to react. *Because they don't see the real you, they can't give you what you need.*

Karen was experiencing this every day.

I'm sure you've seen her, the ice-cold woman. She's colder than an Antarctic icepick. She's emotionally cold and seemingly lives without feelings and empathy. Although she can initially do well in business, she fails in all other areas of her life.

Ice-cold women aren't born that way. Babies are always emotionally warm and open to everything. They are bundles of joy. That's how you are supposed to be!

Now ice-cold women, in particular, were often very loving and creative creatures. They were generally *very* sensitive at first. But upon coming in contact with the badness in this world, be that an unloving parent, losing a loved one, disrespectful boyfriends, or the unfaithfulness of a lover, they decided to become cold as a defensive strategy. It seemed safer that way.

A woman like this believes if she shields off her heart so no one can touch it, she will avoid pain. Better to have no feelings at all, than get hurt!

She is wrong. Dead wrong. This strategy always backfires. The pain she will avoid is severely dwarfed in comparison to the love and affection she will miss out on.

The high-value woman loves fully. She's not afraid to get hurt. She gets hurt too, plenty of times! The big difference between the high- and not-so high-value woman is that the former is not afraid of negative emotions. She *owns* those feelings when they come; she embraces them and then decides what her best course of action is *despite* the emotions she's feeling.

When it comes to matters of the heart, the high-value woman uses "hurt" as a simple radar to decide who should get some of her lovin' and who shouldn't.

Your mind is designed to avoid pain and seek pleasure. The challenge is that, for your survival, your mind avoids pain *much* more than it will seek out pleasure. A simple example will clarify why: just imagine the most beautiful waterfall in a warm jungle. It's a welcoming present since you're soaking in sweat. The air is

84

filled with butterflies, and the pond with the waterfall is so inviting. It would be such a pleasure to take a dive on this warm day, if it weren't for the three crocodiles that were lurking in the background, waiting for the first animal to take a plunge. Not to mention the anaconda quietly sitting at the bottom of the pond, and the school of hungry piranhas hiding behind one of the water plants with a huge grin on their faces. It's because of situations like these that we stay hesitant and skeptic when there is pleasure to be had. Our mind continuously looks for possible dangers, and this comes in handy quite often, especially in the jungle.

Unless it doesn't serve us. And when you've been bitten before, when you've been hurt by someone—a lover, a colleague, a friend, or a relative—your brain will try to avoid that pain at all costs. It's natural. Emotional pain feels just as painful as getting punched in the stomach, as psychologist Matthew Lieberman from UCLA proved in an interesting study.[12] Social pain follows the same pathways in the brain as physical pain does.

Now as you know, the high-value woman doesn't follow her natural instincts without questioning them. It's not because she feels an emotion that she follows up on it. She always uses her emotional intelligence to take a step back and decide: is this emotion serving me?

Is this jealousy I'm feeling serving me? Is it good for the long term?

---

[12] Does Rejection Hurt? An fMRI Study of Social Exclusion
https://www.researchgate.net/publication/9056800_Does_Rejection_Hurt_An_fMRI_Study_of_Social_Exclusion

Is this anger I'm feeling assisting me? Will it help me in the long term if I act out and get angry now? Is it good for future me?

Is this love I'm feeling helping me? Am I falling for the right guy or am I blinded by love?

Is the fact that I want to shield myself off aiding me? Am I under attack by real piranhas? Is there a problem now, right now, that I need my shields for?

Is this fear I'm feeling serving me? Should I put my defenses up or am I reacting because of a past experience and will I possibly miss out on a great adventure?

Ice-cold women *always* take a defensive stance. They are so afraid to get hurt, that while avoiding the bad, they prefer to not experience the good—any of it, for some. It's collateral damage, and they're fine with it. That makes sense when that pain would represent a physical danger. It's pointless to jump out of a sailboat to take a pleasant and refreshing swim with your inflatable dolphin when you've just seen a shark giving you the eye. Yet, so many women got hurt emotionally one day and consequently decide to skip a lot of the pleasures life has to offer altogether.

This happens in their romantic life when they decide men are not to be trusted. I can assure you that indeed, men *are* not to be trusted until they prove otherwise. But the high-value woman still goes for it. She prefers to get hurt rather than to miss out. She knows it is part of the game of life.

Friendships can be tricky too. Most ice-cold women don't have a lot of them. The ice-cold woman's guard is up so much that other people can't reach her authentic self. It's tough being charismatic and authentic when you're wearing a mask *and* a huge impenetrable shield. Other people just stop inviting her because she's no fun to be around.

Her coldness hurts her equally at work. Even though it can serve her business wise, she never feels accepted by her colleagues and feels isolated.

This may be something you seemingly don't suffer from since I'm sure you are a warm and loving woman, but I beg to differ. You do come in contact with this law. The problem of the ice-cold woman is not that she is cold! She is often warm and loving on the inside just like everyone else, but she wears a mask. That mask is the core issue that everyone can suffer from.

Everyone is wearing a mask at different moments. Whenever you adapt in an effort to not upset someone, whenever you try to be liked, whenever you say "yes" when you really want to say "hell no!" you're wearing a mask. And the world cannot respond to you in its most favorable way when you do.

When you wear a mask, neither the people you come in contact with, nor the opportunities you get, will feel compatible with who you are. It's because of the mask! Walk around with an actual ski mask for twenty-four hours, and you will see exactly what I mean. And even though it's obvious there, people still respond to the persona displayed through the invisible masks people wear. Given that a mask doesn't represent who you truly are, others will often be treating you the wrong way.

I cannot drive this point home enough.

Take off your mask as much as you can. Allow yourself to get hurt, to learn from your mistakes, and then to move on with an open heart. That is the best way to get what you want and for others to respond just the way you need.

Flirtation, One of the Most Powerful Weapons

Flirtation is one of the many arts women are really good at, but they don't always use to the fullest. Some *only* use it when they are on the lookout for a man and once they have one, flirtation gets stored in a box. Yet, it can be used for so much more.

Picture an emotionally weak woman with very low self-esteem; let's say she's at a networking event.

How would she behave?
How would she walk?
How would she talk?

Two images might come to mind. The most prevalent one is that of the woman who's carefully watching her words, not making too much eye contact, and not speaking up. By the end of the evening, most people didn't know she was there, even though she stood right next to them.

There's nonetheless another form that she might appear in. She might be the loud woman who raises her voice and grabs the attention in an effort to feel important. When she walks by you would know, just because of the unavoidable ear damage you would suffer. By the end of the evening, everyone noticed she was there. The question is, did anyone care? Would anyone enjoy seeing her again?

loud

Now picture a self-confident, high-value woman. She's present at the same networking event.

How would she behave?
How would she walk?
How would she talk?

She's different. She's charismatic. She talks, but she doesn't raise her voice. She doesn't try to appear important. When she walks, she does so in her own feminine way. When she talks, she has something to say and some value to add to the conversation. Not because she wants to be important, but she wants *the other people* to feel important.

When the loud woman with low self-esteem talks to you, you might say afterward, "She believes she's very important." When the high-value woman talks to you, you'll say, "She made *me* feel very important."

Guess who people love to be around the most?
Guess what woman has had the most fun by the end of the evening?

The high-value woman understands the art of flirtation. She doesn't use it overtly. She's not a bimbo, after all. But flirting she does, often. Not just with men, mind you. She can flirt with everyone. When she turns it on, everyone feels special including other women!

You might think, "Um Brian, isn't that just people pleasing? Isn't she seeking approval then?" Good question. No, of course, she isn't. She doesn't try to get anything from anyone, definitely not their approval. She does it because it makes *her* feel good.

She comes first.

It's never about manipulation and never comes across as insincere. When she says something, she means it.

You may have noticed that true charismatic and magnetic people don't want anything from you. They're not seeking out your compliments, your approval, or anything else. They have a way of making you feel good, regardless of how you will respond. They give without expecting *or needing* anything in return, and their energy is unchanged by your reactions.

When charismatic people give a compliment, it never comes across as sleazy or with a hidden agenda. They actually mean it! Kindness is very high in their mission statement. Interestingly enough, "having clear boundaries and not seeking to be liked" will always be near the top of their list as well. That's what makes them charismatic instead of people pleasers.

Always remember the golden rule: the person who depends the least on what the other person thinks will automatically attract the other one. And as is the case in every negotiation, the person who depends the least on the outcome will always have the power and the upper hand. And even though that effect will be the strongest in romantic relationships, it doesn't end there. It works everywhere. The art of flirting is not just meant to find a mate.

Flirtation is all about having fun in a non-weak way. I'll explain. Let's look at the difference between bad and good flirtation first. A woman with low self-esteem likes a man and wants to flirt with him, so she says, "I really like you. You're attractive." What she hopes for is that the man will return the compliment so *she* can feel good. When she says, "Oh that's a nice purse," she hopes the woman she complimented will return the favor with a "Thanks, I like your blouse." She *needs* something from the people she flirts with. The people she uses this upon know this all too well, sadly for her. Her compliments and attention never feel sincere.

A high-value woman finds a man interesting—she doesn't like him yet, he'll have to prove his worth first—and she wants to flirt with him. She says, "That's a nice jacket. It shows that you've

90

been working out." She smiles, and her eyes communicate that she's having fun. She doesn't want anything in return from that man. If he's into her, he'll play along. If he's not, that's fine too. When she says, "That's a nice purse," she says so as a gift to the woman she complimented *and* because she really likes the purse. She flirts just for fun.

So how do other people know the difference between bad and good flirting when it's used upon them? It's in our instincts. I'm sure you've felt it when someone was complimenting you or flirting with you just to get something in return. It results in a very oppressive feeling, comparable to getting an unwanted hug from an uncle who believes that deodorant and toothpaste are just some countries in Europe.

Whereas men need to learn it, good flirtation is in your natural instincts as a woman. Many of my friends have daughters between the ages of three and eight years old. It astounded me how soon they started to flirt, often as soon as they were two-year-olds. I don't think they have flirting classes in kindergarten, so these are innate feminine powers. They flirt with their daddy when they want to get something their mommy would disapprove of. They even flirt with me when I'm visiting, and they're good at it!

When you enter into your true flirtatious zone, you'll be energetic, radiant, feminine, enthusiastic, and powerful. On top of what you'll feel inside energy-wise, flirtation changes other people's behavior too; especially that of men, although that's not news to you.

My sister once had to park her car on the ramp of a dangerous turn on a busy highway. The gas meter had been showing "empty" for a while, but she figured her car would last long enough to fill it up at the gas station near her house. Well, it didn't last. When two cops pulled over, ready to give her a ticket and reprimand her, she did what any woman should do: she turned on her flirtation in a *very* subtle way. Long story short, those cops gave her a ride to the next gas station with sirens and flashing lights and escorted her to the front of the line so she didn't have to wait. Then they brought her back, with sirens again, and even helped her fill up the car and get it started. Few men would be able to get that kind of presidential treatment.

Flirtation communicates so much to others. It shows them that you are satisfied with who you are, that you're feeling alive and full of energy, and that you're happy. There is no fear, no doubt, no stress because these are incompatible with true flirtation. That's why it's so attractive to other people! It's pure sassiness, and everyone loves to be around that energy.

Everyone is attracted to other people having fun, as scientific studies show time and time again.[13]

If you happen to be introverted and shy, you'll still be able to use this concept. Flirtation is not about being loud, super social, overtly sexual, or direct. It's an internal game. It makes you radiate from the inside out. You could be flirting with someone while not saying a word or while having a normal conversation. The flirtatious internal energy strengthens your self-confidence; it makes you happy to be there, wherever that is. It's an energy.

---

[13] Garry Chick, Careen Yarnal, Andrew Purrington, Play and Mate Preference, Testing the Signal Theory of Adult Playfulness, http://www.journalofplay.org/sites/www.journalofplay.org/files/pdf-articles/4-4-article-chick-play-and-mate-preference.pdf and Humor ability reveals intelligence, predicts mating success, and is higher in males, Gill Greengross, Geoffrey Miller, Intelligence, Volume 39, Issue 4, July–August 2011, Pages 188-192

It's not overtly visible. Other people just feel it when they are around you.

A quick way to see your own flirtation in action is to stand in front of a mirror and to then think of something that delights you! Think of all the details and visualize you partaking in whatever it is that excites you. Visualize the experience, the sights, the sounds... everything.

Or, while you're looking in the mirror, think of a naughty secret you know about someone that you're not supposed to be aware of. Before long, your eyes will start to light up, you'll get a subtle smirky smile, and you'll start to radiate an attractive energy.

Please try this exercise so you can *see* it!

"Stop, Brian," you may still think. "I don't need to 'flirt', I already have a great man." Or "I don't want to flirt, I don't want to attract *more* men. I'm already being whistled at enough as I walk around, you have no idea! What planet are you from?"

Well, Mars apparently, but I'll explain. It's true, when you are being magnetic, you will not only attract the high-quality metals but also the scraps. Nevertheless, flirtation is not *just* for attracting men. Not at all in fact! That's just one of the many uses. Flirtation is about making you feel like a woman. True flirtation is not a masculine thing; it's what makes a woman feminine. It will make you feel great and a lot of people who come in contact with you in the process will benefit from it as well. When you shut down your flirtatious side for any reason, you're shutting down a part of you that makes you a woman. You might think no harm is done, but you will begin to feel it.

I'll never forget a story I once read about Marilyn Monroe, the embodiment of flirtation. She was walking around in New York

City with a photographer named Ed Feingersh. Everybody who walked by didn't notice her, not even as she was standing in a packed subway wagon. She was not wearing a wig, a mustache, or any other kind of disguise. She was very recognizable, but Norma Jean had simply turned off that what made her Marilyn Monroe. When the photographer confronted her with what was happening, she said, "You would like to see Marilyn?" and then she switched it on. Her posture changed, her eyes started to radiate, her smile came alive, and not before long people started to notice her. "It's Marilyn Monroe!" they yelled in a frenzy. Nothing had changed besides her flirtation being turned on.

It's what makes women come alive.

Feminine

One of the high-value women I once met gave me an instruction manual on how to turn it on, should you need it. She said, "Whenever I want to fire it up, even if I just want to flirt with the barista at the coffee shop, I start to think about something that excites me. I might start to think about how sexy I believe my legs are, or I remember a time I fell in love and was flooded by butterflies. If it's a cute guy I might think about what he would look like in his Tarzan suit. I picture something that excites me, and that makes me feel alive and feminine."

This may not be news to you, but all of the high-value women I interviewed after learning about this subject myself confirmed that people, all people, behave differently around them when they turn it on. People go out of their way to say hi, they serve them first, they remember their name, they make sure to invite them whenever they're hosting a party or a dinner—they just want to be around them. Why wouldn't they?

Everyone loves to be around someone who knows how to feel good in their own skin, someone who enjoys herself, somebody who feels fantastic. A ridiculous concept, isn't it? Especially coming from a man, I know.

I *have* been coaching women for a long time. This works remarkably well!

Stay in touch with that flirtatious girl inside of you whether you're single or have been married for decades. She'll be stoked every time you let her out.

Let's Talk About Hormones

Ah, the big enigma for most men: trying to understand why a woman can be so influenced by her menstrual cycle, menopause, or anything else that changes her hormones. Men wonder why women seem to be on emotional rollercoasters, having ups and downs, when men themselves are as emotionally flat as a pancake.

The difference between men and women not only originates from their different energies, it also arises from the male dominant hormone, testosterone, and the female dominant hormone, estrogen. In fact, testosterone is what gives men their masculine energy. It's the hormone that makes them ambitious and gives them the will to win. Likewise, it makes them want to fight when needed, want to succeed, want to do just about anything that makes them masculine instead of feminine.

Both men and women have a mix of estrogen and testosterone, with testosterone being more abundant in men.

As a woman, there will be times when you will benefit from a testosterone-shot to instantly boost your power. Testosterone has many positive side effects. The fact that it greatly reduces unconscious stress and anxiety is one of them.[14]

---

[14] Testosterone Reduces Unconscious Fear but Not Consciously Experienced Anxiety: Implications for the Disorders of Fear and Anxiety. Jack van Honk, Jiska S. Peper, and Dennis J.L.G. Schutter
https://www.researchgate.net/profile/Jiska_Peper/publication/7803720_T estosterone_Reduces_Unconscious_Fear_but_Not_Consciously_Experienced_ Anxiety_Implications_for_the_Disorders_of_Fear_and_Anxiety/links/0c9605 1540a15200d2000000/Testosterone-Reduces-Unconscious-Fear-but-Not-Consciously-Experienced-Anxiety-Implications-for-the-Disorders-of-Fear-and-Anxiety.pdf

Amy Cuddy, professor of social psychology at Harvard, has found through her research that taking a power pose—standing like Superman or sitting with your feet up on the desk and taking up a lot of space—for as little as two minutes, significantly raised the testosterone levels in the study subjects, making them feel more powerful. The side effect was that it also significantly decreased cortisol, the stress hormone.

If you ever find yourself in a situation where you could benefit from some "male" power to speak up, to be assertive, or to simply stand your ground firmly, load up on some testosterone by using a power pose. Stand like Superman did. Head up straight, chest forward, arms as wide as possible, and hands against your sides, and hold this position for two minutes to let the hormonal shift take place, as proven by the scientific research at Harvard.[15] Do it in the elevator as you're riding up, in the restrooms, or wherever you can charge up your testosterone batteries.

If you cannot be alone and you find yourself in a situation where Superman's presence would be frowned upon, just try to take up more space. Don't sit like a woman this time, sit like a man (no crossed legs, arms as wide as possible, even if it means having your arm on the headrest of the chair next to you). If you're standing, position your legs a bit wider, lean forward, and if possible, put your hands on a table with your arms apart.

Power poses can help with a variety of problems. Studies have shown that higher testosterone also helps to stop excessive

---

[15] Amy J. C. Cuddy, Caroline A. Wilmuth, and Dana R. Carney, The Benefit of Power Posing Before a High-Stakes Social Evaluation, https://dash.harvard.edu/bitstream/handle/1/9547823/13-027.pdf?sequence=1

worrying and overthinking. [16] Combine that with the lower levels of cortisol from a power pose and you're golden.

A bit of masculine energy can come in handy every now and then. However, never turn off your feminine energy since that may turn you into the ice-cold woman from a few chapters back.

---

[16] https://www.ncbi.nlm.nih.gov/pubmed/22972022

The Formula for Unstoppable Confidence

Nobody likes pain, well, aside from people who like dungeons, leather whips, and grown men dressed as babies asking for a spanking—but that's a whole different ballgame. As previously demonstrated, both your body and your brain will do what they can to avoid getting hurt. That's fine when it comes to not licking the cookie dough off the mixer spatulas when they're still spinning, but not OK when you're trying to avoid emotional pain in the process.

What I'm about to explain will sound very simple, yet it took me over a decade to uncover that *this* is one of the more important secrets of all of the high-value women and men I've ever studied or interviewed.

Drumroll...

The trick in life is not minding when it hurts. I know that may seem anticlimactic. But when you let this sink in, you're about to get all sorts of AHA moments.

Some people go to great lengths to avoid getting hurt:

- They stay with the wrong partner because they fear the hurt that comes from being alone again.

- They keep working for the same company, even though they're unhappy there. Burning that bridge, moving on, and the incertitude will hurt.

- They don't state their boundaries to others because they fear the hurt that will come from the possible rejection or conflict that may follow.

- They don't start their own company because they want to avoid the hurt that comes from failing and having to return to a normal job.

- They keep complaining about "where is this going?" because they don't want to get hurt later on.

Will these indeed prevent them from getting hurt? Or might it be possible that they will end up getting hurt even *more*?

Everyone gets hurt; it's unavoidable.

The big trick in life really is not minding when it hurts. Those who don't mind are truly *alive* and have experiences that the fearful group will forever be deprived of.

Everything that's worth living for can get you hurt. It comes with the territory. Every time you dive into a relationship, you *will* get hurt! There's no possible way to avoid it. Whether you play it safe or not, whether you act like a high-value woman or not, whether you found a good guy or not, you will get hurt at times. Relationships hurt, even the best ones.

When you want a good career or start your own company, you will get hit. There will be obstacles that will keep you up all night. There will both be good and very tough times. There will be competitors that will try to eat your sandwich as soon as you look away. It always comes with the territory.

The group of people that avoids getting hurt gets hurt too. Their challenge is that because of their evasive actions, they *will* avoid all the highs in life while *still* experiencing the lows.

High-value people don't avoid getting hurt. They are not afraid to be vulnerable. They live by the great Nazi camp survivor and famous psychologist Victor Frankl's statement: "Pain is inevitable, suffering is optional. It's a choice."

They go all-in, and they deal with the challenges and the pain that come their way. They are not reckless, of course, they take emotionally intelligent and calculated risks, but they never avoid getting hurt.

Many scientific studies show that confidence—pure core confidence—is built when you take action *and* when that action comes with a certain risk or may cause you to fail.[17] Core confidence is always built upon the risks you took and survived.

A toddler would never become confident in walking had she or he not taken the risk to fall and fail first. It is the risk taking, failing, and seeing that the sun still comes up the very next day that births the confidence.

And risk taking doesn't mean jumping off a plane with a faulty parachute betting that it will still open. It can be as small as speaking up during a meeting even though your answer may be imperfect and may evoke some funny looks. Or seeing a sexy stranger at a networking event, walking over, and engaging in

---

[17] https://www.ncbi.nlm.nih.gov/pubmed/22512502 (The impact of self-confidence on the compromise effect.) https://hbr.org/2011/04/how-to-build-confidence, https://www.ncbi.nlm.nih.gov/pubmed/27474142 (A Multilab Preregistered Replication of the Ego-Depletion Effect.) https://www.ncbi.nlm.nih.gov/pubmed/26197942 (Physical self-confidence levels of adolescents: Scale reliability and validity), https://www.ncbi.nlm.nih.gov/pubmed/21158259 (Leaders, self-confidence, and hubris: what's the difference?)

conversation. Or shopping in the supermarket, picking out two melons, walking over to a gentleman and asking, "What do you think of my melons?" OK, maybe not that last one—but you get the gist of it. All of the above will make you feel alive when you succeed, *even* when you fail.

Life is not about succeeding all the time. Failure is just as necessary as the air you breathe. Those who avoid failures, achieve nothing, by definition.

The point is this: risk getting hurt emotionally. Risk getting rejected. That's the fertile soil where all self-confidence flourishes. And when these "risks" don't feel like risks anymore, move out of your comfort circle and onto bigger things. Keep moving outside of your comfort zone, so you can get comfy feeling uncomfortable.

So many people spend their entire lives living in the tiny comfort zone they became accustomed to. They never step outside of it and thus never enlarge it. Our comfort circles are elastic. We need to keep pushing the limits if we want to grow them. Offer yourself up to give an important presentation, lead a meeting, take that dance class, apply for that job, start that side business, write that book even when you don't *have* to—go for it!

Plus, it's when you fail that you learn. I've learned so much more from my failures than I have from my successes, both in my professional and my personal life.

Let's look at *the* most scary thing *any* man can do. Scarier than flossing the teeth of a great white shark: walking up to a woman he likes and introducing himself. God forbid she says something hurtful like, "Get lost, you creep!" No joke, this is scary as hell to every guy when he first participates in this risky activity. Most men will go to great lengths to avoid any of these types of rejections.

However, some men do face these rejections, get accustomed to them, and get better.

That's how these adventurous men learn that:
- Pickup lines are overrated
- A simple "hello" will often do
- Don't talk about melons
- Be genuinely interested or don't walk over at all...

If a man walked up to three women and succeeded every time, would that make him confident in approaching women? At the surface, it may seem so. But if the fourth woman tells him to take a hike, none of his so-called confidence will be left. He'll be weeping in the corner before you know it. It is not *core* confidence yet because he never got hurt first, he never failed *first*. His confidence will only be built after getting shot down, picking himself up, and still getting another girl's number later.

True confidence is built when you fail, survive, and get better.

Getting What You Want

People who go for what they want and get it have always inspired me. At first, it seemed they had a lot of luck and good old lady fate liked them much more than she liked me.

I was wrong.

The go-getters just "go" a lot more than I did at the time. If you want to win the lottery, you have to play first and probably more than once.

There are two types of people: those who go after what they want and those who wait for permission or for their anxiety to vanish first. That won't happen, because most of what we want is on the other side of fear. Stepping through the fear comes with the territory.

The go-getters try and fail a lot, but at least they try, thus significantly increasing the odds of actually getting something.

The second group is different. They wait for permission, for all the lights to turn green. When you revisit them ten years later, they're often still waiting in the *exact* same position, stuck in the same perpetual loop.

We've already dealt with fear holding you back. This is different; it's not necessarily about fear. It's about waiting until the lights turn green. About holding on until there's a sign that it's OK to execute the idea you've had.

Let's say Jane has always dreamed of writing a book. She has a story she's been thinking of, but she hasn't written down a single word. She's waiting for the kids to be older or wants to find a good boyfriend first. Or she has a sick mother and wants to take care of her first. The lights aren't green at the moment.

Will they ever be?

Or what about Fonda? She has dreamed of visiting Australia ever since she was a kid. She hasn't yet, because the flight alone would take her more than twenty-four hours. The jet lag would be enormous, making a stay of at least two weeks a necessity. She has the money for the trip; that's not the problem. Time is her real challenge. There are plenty of things she *has* to do every week, and she has no idea where to clear up two or more weeks on her calendar. She decides to wait until her life is a bit less hectic. The lights aren't green now.

Will they ever be?

Briana has a similar problem. She's been planning to open a little online shop to sell some of her homemade jewelry. Briana has been designing jewelry ever since she was a little girl, and she's really talented. When she spoke about her idea of opening that shop, people told her they doubted her. They said, "You can't ask money for that. Who's going to pay for your jewelry when they can order it super cheap on one of those Chinese sites?" or "You won't be able to combine that with your day job!" and the best one of all, "Have you even studied to be a designer? Didn't you study to be an accountant?"

Briana thinks these nosy-parkers might be right. It's true that there's a ton of competition out there, and it might fail. And even though she's been designing alluring pieces for over a decade, she indeed never finished a formal study course on designing. She decides to keep doing what other people do and instead of working on her shop at night after work, she continues to watch *The Real Housewives*, just like her friends do. The lights aren't green, and the permission is clearly not given for her to venture into her dreams.

Do these stories sound familiar?

Now ask yourself the following questions:

1. What if Thomas Edison had been waiting for all the proverbial lights to turn green ... as he was inventing the very light bulb and was failing miserably at first?

2. What if Martin Luther King had decided to say, "I have a dream ... but I don't want to talk about it yet" because the lights weren't green? I can assure you they weren't at the time.

3. What if Sara Blakely who invented Spanx would have listened to the first storeowners who turned her down? What if she had decided to put her ideas back in the fridge after "important people" didn't get why Spanx would be handy?

4. What if Erika Mitchell, a very normal housewife and a mother of two teenage sons, had waited *any* longer before she finally wrote and published her book? *Fifty Shades of Grey* became one of the best-selling erotic novels of all time, yet she was nowhere near a famous writer beforehand. All she had written were some self-published fan fiction books that weren't really successful.

You don't need to wait for permission or the lights to turn green. You don't need to wait for friends and family to give an "all clear" when you want to go after one of your dreams. You don't need to wait for your loved ones to approve of the adventure you want to embark upon. You don't even need to wait for them to understand it all. And you definitely don't need to wait for your anxiety or hesitance to pass first.

It's better to shoot for the stars and miss, than to aim for the mud and make it.

It's your life. This is not the dress rehearsal. This is the only shot you have. And even though not all lights are green, they may never get greener than they are right now.

"But I'm not a risk taker, Brian," some women tell me. Says who?

"Yeah but my family wouldn't approve, we play it safe," you might say. Good for them! But following your dreams isn't about risking your life or betting all of your savings. That would be foolish indeed. Common sense is always useful. It's about the small ideas that pop up in your head, the "I should..." that you then immediately dismiss because the lights ... aren't green.

It's about writing that book, taking that vacation, visiting that long-lost friend, taking a short trip, learning that new language, going for that walk in nature, learning that new skill you wish you mastered, starting that side business that doesn't require massive investments, or working on any of your other ideas that make your heart beat a little bit faster when you think of it.

It's about what matters to you, because you come first.

When you take an honest look at yourself, how many well-meaning people who are still stuck in the same position they have been in for decades have smashed your ideas to pieces? People who would love for you to stay there too, so they can have some company and feel a tiny bit better about themselves. Those are not the people you should ever take advice from.

For most of the things I've succeeded at, I've had plenty of people tell me why I shouldn't have started. If I had listened to them I would have missed out on a lot of successes. Failures too, of course, because they are just as important. That's when you learn! There's no success without failure, no learning to walk without falling, so I personally never regret my failures either.

You can't ever get the relationship that fulfills you without some trial and error. Many errors, as you will undoubtedly have experienced. You can't get the job that gives you pleasure without going through some work places that make you miserable. Success is always built upon many failures. It has taken successful people a long time and a lot of failures to become an "overnight" success.

The lights never *get* green. The permission doesn't come from outside of us; it comes from within. Give yourself the permission to go after what you want. Nobody else will. You come first.

Why Men Are Stealing Your Power...and *How* They Do It

This is an important chapter. I'm sure you're not living on women's island where no men are allowed. Whether you live with one or not, there are men you'll come into contact with. Those in the supermarket who want to talk about melons, superiors and underlings in the workplace, silly whistlers in the streets, and the most dangerous type of all: the one you have feelings for.

If I asked you to look back at the past ten to twenty years of your life, how many hours have you spent worrying about men? You can pick anything from the list below; please check all that apply:

- "Does he like me?"

- "Why doesn't he call? He told me he would call!"

- "How come he doesn't appreciate it any longer when I...?"

- "How come _____ became more important than spending time with me?"

- "I start to get the feeling that I'm the only one who takes care of..."

- "I've asked him X times to _____, and he still didn't do it. Is that what brain-dead looks like?"

- "What's the deal with forgetting important dates?"

- "Why can't he just listen, without always coming up with solutions?"

- "When is he going to ask me out? I think I've made it more than clear that I like him."

- "He tells me I need to support him while he's trying to get that promotion at work or as he's starting that new venture, but I have my own stuff to worry about too!"

- "He seemed interested and told me he liked me, so why is he behaving so distant?"

- "Something's off, but he tells me everything is fine."

- "He tells me he's not looking for anything serious, but I have a feeling he may just be lying to himself, maybe he's afraid..."

- "When it comes to making a choice that could benefit my own growth, I'd better make sure it fits *his* plans as well. However, it seems like he's not doing that for me."

- "Why did Bob, of all creatures, get promoted over me? I'm working harder and better..."

This is not an exhaustive list. I could keep going and write a 14,654-page book filled with examples, but I'm sure you get the point. Every time you worry about a guy, be that a love interest or even Bob at work, he's stealing some of your power. It's impossible to be focused and to be growing if your mind keeps wandering off to worry about *him* and what he did or did not do. I know women are great at multitasking, but still...

If this doesn't apply to you and you never have to worry about men, please skip this chapter ... and reach out to me. You may have found the Holy Grail, and I would love to hear more about it!

Chances are you're still reading....

Many women pick the wrong man and stay with him. That first part, picking the wrong guy, is normal. You're probably not hooking him up to a lie detector straight out of the gate. It's impossible to know who you're really dealing with until deep down into the dating stage or even the relationship. The mistake is made when you *stay* with a man who's keeping you from becoming the woman you are.

Now honestly, I can't apportion all the blame to men. There are a lot of good and great men out there. It's easy to have worries about your relationship when you *need* him, when you depend on him, even with the good guys. That's a trap that not only the nice girl steps into. Today's society is still built upon the premise that if you don't have a good man, kids, a house ... well, then something must be wrong with you.

Right....

Let's look at how ridiculous this is. My girlfriend is a successful psychologist and therapist. She meets women each and every day who have everything. To society's standards, they are successful. Yet they are as miserable as a penguin strolling around the hot desert.

Again, there's nothing wrong with looking for a good man, kids, a house—plenty of people are totally fulfilled when they get it right. But it's not meant for everyone and definitely not at all costs. I have met many women who frantically go after the entire list. Not because they want it, they do so because they believe they *should* want it. No good can come from this. This, in my experience, is the prime reason why some women accept mediocre behavior from men. They believe being single is worse than being with a guy who doesn't treat them perfectly right.

Is it *really*?

Some women put all of their energy into finding or keeping *any* guy who checks at least some of the boxes. They *need* him. As a result, these women have become way too dependent on men.

That's not the natural way.

There was a time where men fought to get the attention of a woman. And when I say fought, I'm talking about bloody fights and actual wars with armies and severed limbs. I'm sure you've heard of Troy and other famous men who started battles for the woman they loved. Nowadays, most women have to be happy with a bouquet of flowers and a little note every three years or so. Times have changed.

The human race comes from a time where everyone was living in close-knit groups and communities. Back then women didn't *need* a man. They had lots of love, affection, and connection from other women and the rest of the group they were living in. Single people or couples were not living all alone on their private property, they were always part of a larger group with loads of helping hands and listening ears that were available when needed. They needed a group of people, not *one* man.

Our society is different now, but there is a part in everyone that still longs for that connection to others. A real connection, not the one you get from swiping down social media feeds. This is one of the primal reasons that some women feel perpetually lonely and empty, even when they're in a relationship and have kids.

When you need one man to feel fulfilled, when you try to please one man, when you need the affection of one man to feel like you matter, you're giving away all of your powers. It's a voluntary donation of power.

I'm a big fan of monogamy, don't worry, I'm not advocating building a harem of docile men. However, through my research and experience, I noticed the high-value woman has a specific way to deal with this particular challenge.

She never lays all of her eggs in one basket. Even though her mind and body might scream to "spend as much time with *him* as you can," she won't. And it's that independence that makes her so attractive to most men. It's *because* she doesn't need them that they start to need her. This lasts deep into their marriage as well.

Besides the voluntary donations of power, you need to protect yourself from the man-thieves as well. Not all men are good, as I'm sure you have noticed.

Men can try to steal your power in many ways. Some are conscious acts to keep you under control and emotionally stable; others are simply side effects of the male psyche not always being aligned with that of the woman. Let's see how everything can play out.

In the Dating Stage

The best example is the guy who says he likes a woman and sees a future with her even though he knows all too well she's not the one he wants to grow old with.

Most guys get lonely too. They'd rather be with someone they're not really into than be alone. Some men will be open and honest about this. Sadly, the bad guys out of this group will know exactly what to do to string a woman along. And they will!

However, that's where the weakness of this type of bad boy lies. He knows what to *say*, but his actions will speak louder than words. His behavior will give away his disinterest, and you'll at the very least get a feeling in your gut that something's not right. He'll be investing the absolute minimum into the relationship to still get what he needs.

The high-value woman tries to see through his words and only looks at his actions. When he says, "I really love spending time with you, and I want to keep seeing you," yet he always arrives late on dates, reschedules, or even cancels dates, she will not give him the benefit of the doubt. NEXT!

Always remember that most men show their *best* selves during the dating stage. It will only go downhill from there.

In conclusion, in the dating stage, men try to steal your power by showing flaky behavior that will make you worry about his true intentions. The rule is simple. *If* you have to worry about his true intentions because of his actual behavior, then he's the type of guy who will never allow you to blossom. If you continue with that guy, you should block off some time every day on your calendar marked as "worry time" for the rest of the relationship. You will need it.

In the Relationship Stage and During Marriage

This is a bit trickier. The deeper you get into the relationship, the more it will be important to look out for what's important to you. If you decided to marry a very compassionate and affectionate man, you might not really get in trouble here. Nevertheless, at times he will have his own self-interest in mind when choices are made that include you. That's normal.

114

But the biggest problem here is that men won't be able to support you emotionally, *even* the good guys. Let's find out why.

Honestly, as a guy, I can affirm that it is very hard on us when our girlfriends or wives become emotionally unstable. We don't get it since we don't suffer from hormones as much as women do. Men, on average, *seem* much more emotionally stable than women. However, as I explained in my other books as well, studies show men cannot handle emotions half as well as women can. They're having a lot of trouble handling themselves, let alone the woman they're in a relationship with.

This is not just my personal opinion, nor is it a fad. Men and women *are* different when it comes to how their brain processes information. And to be honest, besides map-reading, women are the clear winners in every single aspect. What men get in physical strength, women get in emotional strength, as proven by science.

In a study that was published in 2013 in the *Proceedings of the National Academy of Sciences*, Ragini Verma (PhD), a professor in the department of radiology at the University of Pennsylvania, described that although men have better motor and spatial abilities, women have superior memory and social cognition skills. This means that women are *designed* to better handle emotions and mental tasks. Women's brains are more efficient.

There, I said it.

And I'm just getting started. Larry Cahill, a professor at the University of California, found another difference between a man and a woman's brain.[18] Men have a more active and bigger amygdala, the part of the brain that regulates instinctive

---

[18] *Scientific American,* October 1st 2012, His Brain and Her Brain

reactions like the fight-or-flight response. Long story short, a man's brain responds *way* more emotionally to stress than a woman's. Stress and emotions give a man the urge to run for safety and find solitude, whereas a woman will want to connect with other people, preferably friends or loved ones, as proven by this study and by reality.

I'm sure you can imagine how incompatible this makes men and women in relationships, especially if there was a heated argument or worse, a fight.

When you want to talk about anything difficult, he comes preprogrammed to run for the hills. You might wonder what's up there, in those hills. I'll tell you: a lot of frightened men.

So science proves time and time again that most men are allergic to emotions, they cannot handle them well. This can make relationships quite difficult and emotionally draining for both parties.

I'm sure that, as a woman, you've already thought: "he doesn't get me" or "he's not really there for me." You are right and totally correct. He does not get you, and he cannot really be there for you. He anatomically cannot. That's, however, not an excuse! He should at least try.

Nevertheless, don't spend too much of your power and attention on it. He cannot physically get to your level of understanding, compassion, and empathy. That's yet another reason why the high-value woman has a lot of true *female* friends she can confide in. These women give her the support network she needs, so she doesn't have to get emotional support from her boyfriend or husband alone.

I want to emphasize again that I am in no way stating that you should cut him too much slack. He should be there for you and give it everything he has, just like you will. But he won't have as much as you, that's all.

A man cannot carry a woman emotionally, just as you'd probably not be able to carry most men physically.

Ever wonder why men always come up with a solution, when all you wanted was to talk or be listened to?

Now you know why. Talking gives them emotions and requires empathy, God forbid, whereas fixing whatever problem you are facing allows them to get on with their lives and be done with it. I'm no different, honestly. And we, men, truly believe we are helping by providing a step-by-step plan instead of listening to what you want to talk about.

In all transparency, my girlfriend has to make a life-changing decision now as I am writing this chapter. A decision that will change her future and will consequently impact mine as well. We have been talking about it for months now, and I have to admit it is draining me. But what's most remarkable is that when I do give her advice, I need to objectively remove myself from the equation since my mind always wonders how this will impact me, me, me. Focusing on what is best for *her* and removing myself from the equation is challenging. I can imagine some men won't go that far.

In conclusion, men will often steal your power because they believe they have to in order to protect themselves. When their woman becomes emotional, they feel bad. When their woman outgrows them, they feel like a failure. When their woman is upset about something, they'll feel like a failure and will try to come up with solutions, when all you needed was a listening ear.

Remember

Even though good men will try to support you, if you want to blossom, make sure you're surrounded by some good female friends who are prepared to listen. Your man, as much as he loves you, won't be physically able to fulfill your needs.

That being said, even your friends need to be carefully picked, as discussed in the next chapter.

Soul-Matching

One of my favorite quotations is from a man named Jim Rohn who said that we are the average of the five people we spend the most time with.

At first, I couldn't get around to believing it. "Who? Me? I am who I am," my ego said. "Other people don't influence my actions, let alone my personality. I'm solid as a rock. No, as a diamond!"

Then my sanity kicked in, and I started thinking:

"How do you feel when someone around you is consistently depressed or in a bad mood?"

"Well, pretty bad."

"How do you feel when you worry about someone you're close to because they are going through a difficult time?"

"Pretty worried. Or guilty if I catch myself *not* worrying about them."

"How do you feel when everyone around you is not ambitious?"

"Pretty complacent myself. Not achieving anything becomes OK."

"On the other hand, how do you feel when you've got a really ambitious close friend?"

"Pretty motivated. I learn from them, and I grow with them. Their motivation and positive energy will be contagious."

"Or what about when someone is energized, smiling, and happy? How does that influence your mood?"

"Like a shot of vitamins..."

As I went back on the timeline that is my own life, I had to conclude that my closest friends and family had had a colossal impact on how I felt, my decisions, actions, and my potential. From the age of about twelve, friends, parents, and other people I was close to tremendously influenced my big life choices. The schools I chose, the discipline and field of study I selected, the clothes I wore, the sports I picked, the way I treated my body, the pool of potential girlfriends I could pick from, the profession I chose, the town where I decided to live, the risks I took and didn't take. They made me see options I was blind to myself, or they shut doors I was about to walk through, that I sometimes should have.

People in your life have a monumental impact on you. It is bigger than anything you can imagine.

The concept is easily explained too. If you play tennis with someone who is a lot better than you, your level will go up. If you play tennis with someone who plays badly, your level will need to go down if you want *any* of the balls returned to you.

I think that's a nice analogy to life. People always adapt to those who surround them, even when they try not to. And most importantly, even when it's not good to do! The people close to you affect the way you think, your values, the decisions you make, and the self-esteem you will feel, *even* if you use all of the emotional intelligence you've got.

Everyone is subjected to this law, but let's look at my favorite woman first: the nice girl. She's the one who's easily influenced

Bad company corrects good behavior

by others. As previously mentioned, the nice girl is "nice" because she wants her partner, boss, colleagues, or whomever to accept her, and she believes she can achieve it by complying to their everyday whims.

That's the wrong approach ... of course.

Nice girls get run over time and time again. Whenever they've picked themselves up from the last bulldozer that plowed them to the ground, the next one hits them. They might end up in dead-end relationships with men who are clearly unable to give them what they deserve (respect, love, affection), or they get stuck in a job that's all about pleasing others and trying to not ruffle any feathers.

What else is the nice girl to do? She might have tried standing up for herself, but then other people got mad or ignored her. That feels even *worse* than the bulldozer.

Deep down, the nice girl believes she is not enough. She doesn't believe she's worth it. And it's not just nice girls who suffer from this predicament.

This is the reason why it is so important to carefully choose who surrounds you because they *will* influence you no matter what.

Look back at your friends in the different stages of your life: childhood friends, then your friends when you were a teenager, when you became a young adult, and so on. These people have strongly influenced your path in life, the choices you've made, the things you did, *and* the things you've missed out on.

As always, I've got scientific proof too. According to psychologists Elaine Hatfield from the University of Hawaii and John Cacioppo of the University of Chicago, people tend to mimic those surrounding them. From the minuscule details like voice tone, nervousness, happiness, to the major life paths like career choices, relationships, and more.

Have you ever felt yourself becoming more nervous when you were around someone who was speaking nervously even though you were totally calm before? Have you ever yawned because someone close to you yawned? I sure have in both occasions.

You may even have heard of the McClintock study. Martha McClintock, a psychologist from Harvard University, was one of the first to discover that women who live together tend to have similar menstrual cycles. And even when some other studies found that they don't always correlate 100 percent, the hormones of the women who live together *did* affect one another. In 2004, another study by McClintock even found that odors from breastfeeding women have effects on the hormonal cycles of childless women.[19] This proves that the people who surround you influence you in ways you cannot even begin to imagine.

Let's just agree upon the fact that other people influence you heavily in a variety of ways. Not just your life partner but everyone you spend a consistent amount of time with every week.

Spend time with people who make you feel better for as much as you can, people you are truly compatible with. Try to distance yourself as much as possible from people who have values or a way of living that's not compatible with your mission statement, with who you are. Their values, attitudes, and habits will start to infect yours.

---

[19] https://www.scientificamerican.com/article/do-women-who-live-together-menstruate-together/

Furthermore, some people are vampires. They latch on and suck you dry. They're worse than a bulldozer because at least you can see and hear that one coming. Energy vampires do it slowly. These are the friends and colleagues who keep going on and on about their own problems. And when it's your time to share an issue you are facing, they immediately put the spotlight back on themselves.

Imagine the people closest to you get the keys to your brain and your emotions. They get to poke around in there, change how you feel, and influence the decisions you make. I'm sure you wouldn't give the keys to your house to some people you *are* giving the key to your emotional well-being.

Pretty challenging, isn't it? As if life isn't difficult enough. Well, good news, as soon as you're mindful about who gets the key, life becomes significantly easier.

How does the high-value woman handle this? First, she decides that she cannot get along with everyone. If she is her true self, some people will disagree with who she is, avoid her, or even criticize her. That hurts; she is human after all. Nevertheless, the high-value woman has made a promise to herself that she will take on that pain whenever it's presented to her. Avoiding that pain would again be adapting to the other person and thus letting him/her influence her course in life. Her personal mission statement cuts through everything.

Being yourself, becoming who you are meant to become, feels so fulfilling that these short moments of pain fade away compared to the true joy of living your own unique life.

The higher of a tree you become, the more wind you will catch. That's never a reason for any tree not to grow.

This means that the high-value woman deliberately chooses people around her who support her. They don't need to agree with everything she does, but they can't try to hold her down or keep her small. If they try to pull her down and have the "crab in a bucket" mentality, she breaks free and leaves them behind. When you put a couple of crabs in a low bucket, there's always a smart one who tries to crawl out. He could easily, but he never succeeds because the other crabs consistently make sure they pull him down again at each attempt.

When you let the vampires and unsupportive people go, new spots open up that can be filled with the right supporters. Everyone in your circle should be rooting for you most of the time, especially the person you're in a relationship with. If that's someone who wants to change you or act differently, you're in for a rough ride. There especially, you need to be accepted and loved for who you are and all that you are not.

When I first met my long-term girlfriend, there was something about her that reeled me in. At first, her looks played an important role, given that I couldn't see her personality yet. But there was something about her. I had already met a lot of women I found attractive, but with her, I went through the agonizing near-death experience of asking her out. As the first few weeks of the relationship passed by, I started to meet her soul. That's the part I truly fell in love with, the only part that matters in the end.

My girlfriend has been seriously ill for months now. All that does is that it makes me love her even more. Her soul hasn't changed. It's still in there, battling to hopefully get better. And I'm trying to stand next to her, fully armed, for as much as I can. I'm rooting for her and would give my life for her.

I've noticed that high-value women often end up in relationships with men who do indeed love the soul of the woman they're with, men who want their soul to become all that it can be. These guys want to be the strong men behind their women. I'm not the exception, of course, and you may have already found such a man. These men don't try to change their woman and especially don't try to tamper with her feminine energy. That would be like buying a dog and asking it to purr like a cat ... good luck with that!

I personally don't believe in there being just *one* soul mate for everyone. But I do believe everyone needs to find someone who's compatible with their own soul. Soul matching is what I like to call it. And that goes for the friends you surround yourself with as well. Everything and everyone you allow to influence your life should match with your soul as much as possible.

Feelings of Guilt and the Danger Behind Them

When young men grow up, they tend to fight, build camps, learn how to protect themselves, try to get stronger, and try to run faster than the next guy. When you look at young boys playing around, you'll often see little gladiators partaking in physical training. They are preparing for fights, setting traps, building a house, and generally taking care of their family. I was building my first tree house with some friends at the age of seven. We set out ingenious traps with nails going through planks that we'd bury upside down under the leaves. We dug out deep pits that we covered up with some twigs and grass. Even Indiana Jones would have had a hard time getting in.

Nobody taught us this. It's in the instincts of every normal man; it's part of *his* inner lion. He's learning how to fight and defend, his primal job as an adult as far as his instincts are concerned.

Most women are different. It's their nature to seek peace and look for the good in everyone. Even though you will find plenty of girls who love to play in the dirt and build forts, when little girls play with their dolls, they are not setting everything up for imminent and bloody warfare or the stinky wild boar that may mess up their mini-kitchen. When little girls run, they do so to see that colorful butterfly from nearby, not to train for the hunt and kill it.

What I've just described sounds like a stark comparison of genders, doesn't it? Yet science has proven these stereotypes time and time again. In two separate experiments both on monkeys and humans, when placed in front of toys, little boys typically went for the balls, cars, and trucks while little girls went for the dolls (*even* the monkeys).[20] Other studies further proved that it's both caused by hormones and the behavioral pre-programmed roles of males and females in society, coming from our evolution. In short: androgen, a class of male hormones to which testosterone belongs, activates a baby's willingness to move and to hunt.[21] These differences appear at a very early age. Another study performed at the City University of London showed that these gender preferences start as early as a couple of months after birth, before there were any effects of socialization. In that study, in the group of babies aged between 9-17 months, the boys went for the ball, the girls for the cooking pot. At such a young age![22]

There are, of course, exceptions to this rule. Some women are petrol heads or like shooting guns. But it is not the norm. According to a group of researchers, these exceptions happen when girls experience high male sex hormone levels while still in the womb. These girls then prefer to have male friends, play with masculine toys, and wish for masculine careers.[23] There's absolutely nothing wrong with that, of course, but it is the

---

[20] Melissa Hines and Gerianne M. Alexander - 2009 - Monkeys, girls, boys and toys: A confirmation Comment on "Sex differences in toy preferences: Striking parallels between monkeys and humans"
https://www.ncbi.nlm.nih.gov/pmc/articles/PMC2643016/

[21] Gerianne M Alexander, Melissa Hines – 2002 - Sex differences in response to children's toys in nonhuman primates (Cercopithecus aethiops sabaeus)
http://www.ehbonline.org/article/S1090-5138%2802%2900107-1/abstract

[22] Brenda K. Todd, John A. Barry, Sara A. O. Thommessen Preferences for 'Gender-typed' Toys in Boys and Girls Aged 9 to 32 Months
https://www.city.ac.uk/news/2016/july/infants-prefer-toys-typed-to-their-gender,-says-study,
http://onlinelibrary.wiley.com/doi/10.1002/icd.1986/full

[23] Prenatal androgens and gender-typed behavior: a study of girls with mild and severe forms of congenital adrenal hyperplasia. Servin A1, Nordenström A, Larsson A, Bohlin G. https://www.ncbi.nlm.nih.gov/pubmed/12760514

exception and not the norm.

Whereas men are designed to hunt and defend, women are designed to look for the good in people, on average. And most women need to get burned at least once before their naiveté will start to diminish.

There is a major nature versus nurture issue at play as well here. *A small percentage of women* is brought up believing in fairy tales. They are looking for the perfect fairy-tale relationship, a wonderfully fulfilling job, and perfect colleagues who never mean any harm. Then, when they come in contact with the real world, they are in for a surprise, especially when their mother taught them to "always be nice." That only makes it worse.

They can go three ways then. They can learn their lessons and toughen up a bit while still remaining open and loving. This is the high-value woman's way. They can shield themselves off and become the ice-cold woman discussed a few chapters back. Or they can remain naive and dive from one disappointment into the next one while not accepting the world as it *is*.

Some women believe the world is this great magical place where everyone should be happy and content. So when someone isn't, when someone is behaving or feeling bad, they will try to fix that person. As if they are an on-call nurse responsible to make others feel better. The unhappy person can be their misery-attracting friend, a colleague, a boss, a husband, a grown child. Somewhere in their minds, they believe it's not only their job to care more and to help these people, they may even feel *responsible* for it.

I'm sure you can sense what a dangerous trap this is. Their entire lives will be built around making other people happy and bringing out the best in others that may not even care themselves. There's no easier way to lose yourself.

I want to be vulnerable with you here. Even though I was building camps as a young gladiator, I believed in fairy tales too. I wanted everyone to be happy. This is something that I have to use my emotional intelligence upon, even to this day. As I was writing the previous chapter on my deck, the neighbor's cat came by for a visit. She's the most interesting cat I've ever seen. Last week she caught a dragonfly, mid-air, while jumping from a tree. When she comes by, I play with her. I throw a stick away, and she gets it for me. I'm dead serious; this is not a normal cat. Now today I was in the midst of passionately writing for you, my lunch was heating up on the stove and I had no time for her. As I closed my laptop and went inside to check on my food, I felt guilty for only petting the cat a couple of seconds.

It gets worse. Last week, I was trimming the bush and felt sorry for my hedge. There she was, trying to reach the sun again after the last trim, and I kept preventing her from ever achieving her goals time and time again.

I blame happy-ending fairytales. It's not my job to make the neighbor's cat or my hedge constantly happy! Yet some of my thoughts believe it is. I luckily know how to dismiss those thoughts now, but that wasn't always the case. As a teenager, I was the nicest of nice guys, trying to please everyone I came in contact with. It nearly killed my soul.

I know I've already said it, but I want to drive this home as much as I can. It is never your job to make other people happy. Aside from your own kids and pets, it is not your job to care for others. You can choose to care and to make someone happy, but it is never your *responsibility*. You needn't feel guilty when you can't.

But that doesn't mean you won't feel the guilt. And just as with the emotions of anxiety and jealousy, you will often need to use your emotional intelligence to decide the emotion is wrong. Take the guilt with you and don't change your actions, it will flow away.

When you believe in fairy tales, you not only want everyone to feel perfectly happy, you often believe there's something good in everyone you meet. That may very well be the case, but here too it is never your responsibility to get it out of them unless you are their actual therapist, teacher, or parent.

Feel free to care and help others! Just know it is not something to feel guilty about when you can't.

You come first.

And this is a very important concept with remarkable effects on your empowerment. People all need to find the middle between "fight for and defend our souls" and the "let's have a cozy tea party so we can all be friends."

How do you feel when you've just disappointed someone? Does it give you a pit in your stomach? Or at least an uneasy feeling? What do you do with that feeling?

As a nice-guy teenager, I couldn't stand it. When someone was disappointed in me, I changed my actions to make him or her happy again. I needed the confirmation that they were all right, that everything was all right between us. Not *just* because I was seeking their approval, mind you. I most importantly wanted to get rid of that feeling in my stomach. I couldn't handle the emotion of guilt.

Conflict with others made me feel very uneasy. But all my pleasing and trying to see the good in others was wearing me down fast. Aside from the anxiety I had, I started to suffer from the chronic fatigue syndrome. Why wouldn't I? I was trying to care about *everyone* I came in contact with. Even people I would never meet again.

Here too, I needed to learn to deal with that feeling of guilt. Not by taking it away and by changing my behavior, but by embracing it and considering it a part of life. Most importantly, by not changing my actions when I felt it! Guilt, for nice people, is a bad advisor.

It's not your job to please everyone. It's not your job to keep searching for the good in someone when they have deliberately hurt your feelings. It's your job to let go of all of that and to go for your mission, even when that means you'll disappoint others.

At this very moment, I have exactly 314 unanswered emails in my inbox from people who want something from me ASAP. It was my pleasure to choose to ignore them so I could spend time working on this book. This is more important to me. And I'm still caring (about you, in this case). It doesn't make me egocentric or emotionally cold.

I come first in my life, as you should come first in yours.

Standing Up for Yourself, the Non-negotiable Way

Other people will continuously try to change you. They will look for your boundaries and see what they can get away with. When you buy a puppy, he'll test you to see what's allowed and what's not. "Can I bite the couch to pieces? Wow, those are nice shoes, must eat them!" When you have a baby, your child will test you and see what's allowed and what's not. When you get a man, he too will test you and see what's allowed and what's not.

And there's nothing wrong with that. They all consider what's important to them and test how much you want to go along with it. It's the natural way. Nevertheless, these are the very moments where we'll need to protect our self and our boundaries. Moreover, some people will not have good intentions and will try to change us through manipulation and other tactics.

Don't let anyone who wants you to be something you're not prevent you from blossoming. Not at home, not a work, not in your family life.

It's as if someone planted rose seeds. But when the first rose starts to bloom that person thinks, "What? This doesn't look like a tulip! I want a tulip!" He or she tears off that first young flower, and the next one, and the next one because they all tend to look like a rose and not a tulip. That rose will never blossom. You must never be that rose!

My sister is a successful lawyer and when she was working as an intern for a huge law firm, her (male) bosses tried to treat her and the other interns like cattle. One Friday at 4:30, her boss smacked a bulky folder filled with papers on her desk. With a serious look on his face, he said, "This is an important case. We need you to go through all of these documents by Monday morning. Try to find anything that helps us strengthen our position." He turned around, ready to walk out of her office. The order had been given, so his job was done.

What he hadn't seen coming was my sister's calm reply. "That will not be possible," she said. "I'm going away for the weekend. I need to recharge my batteries." She had booked a weekend getaway with her boyfriend, something that she really needed since most of her time was spent in the city.

Her boss turned around, visibly getting into uncharted territory. Disobeying a direct order? Nobody had ever committed that kind of sacrilege before.

"Um. No. You are an intern here. You work for me! You need to get this done by Monday," her boss replied with an even harsher look on his face and a strict tone of voice that made it clear this was not a negotiation. It was evident he believed his manipulation would work based on how it must have previously worked on others.

"No, I really won't do it. This weekend is important to me. I cannot get this done by Monday. I *can* start working on it first thing Monday morning if you want," my sister replied, still without raising her voice.

Her boss, on the other hand, was becoming really agitated. His face turned all red, and a vein could have popped anytime. He came back with, "All of the other interns are here 16 hours a day, and they work weekends too." He started to look like a toddler who lost his lollipop.

"With all due respect, then you might want to give it to *them*. If I'm not allowed to recharge my batteries so I can give you my everything five days a week, then this may not be the right place for me to work," my sister calmly replied.

My sister knew she was good at her job. The other interns did spend more hours at the office, but my sister's work got good reviews. That said, she was not bluffing. She knew she could get fired on the spot, and that would have been fine. She refused to shut up her lioness and deviate from her mission statement because she had seen what it had done to our mother, who had a really hard time at work for decades.

This event was more than ten years ago. Her boss eventually apologized for acting like a fool (even though he continued to act like one countless times), promoted her a couple of months later, and she now works for one of the top five law firms in the world.

Every now and then, it will be important to stand up for yourself and put someone else back in line, even when it involves someone you look up to or someone who seemingly controls part of your future.

If you had been a fly on the wall during this conversation, is *this* how you would have thought it would turn out?

It isn't to most people. They're too afraid to stand up for themselves because they visualize impending doom. My sister's boss could have easily fired her with the flick of a finger. But he didn't. I'm proud to call my sister one of the high-value women in my life never afraid to use her power and tell me about it afterward.

She never ever muted herself during her entire career. She almost never works weekends, and she even has Thursday afternoons off to pick up the kids from school and spend some quality time with them while working for a top law firm. She's not that special. Her inner voice also said things like, "Well, I shouldn't go away this weekend because all of the other interns work as well."

There will always be a gazillion excuses to not do what's important to you. You can never shut down the negative voice that comes up with these excuses. But you don't have to!

Can you see what my sister did in this example? How she solved the problem? She employed her *masculine* energy to protect her feminine energy.

Remember, female energy is about teamwork, working together, softness, niceness, caring, and all that is feminine. That's the energy that would *not* have helped her here. She was in a war zone under attack by someone who believed he was a God.

Male energy is about strength, vigor, decisiveness, action, ambition, and crushing your opponent to smithereens. It's about figuratively kicking her boss in the nuts so he changes his tune, which he did in the end.

High-value women know how to use their male energy in such a way that it never dominates their female energy, yet they can use all of its pure force whenever needed. They're all feminine and soft until they are not.

This is one of the advantages women have in the workplace. Most men can only use masculine energy, whereas women can use all of the powers of their feminine energy (which makes them much better leaders) and top it off with some masculine force when needed.

That's what my sister did. Her female energy wanted to go for walks in nature, spend time with her boyfriend (now the father of her children), and take time to relax. She used her male energy to be really decisive and draw the line in the sand *so clearly* that her boss could not miss it. There was no softness or weakness in her sentences and actions. She wasn't asking for his approval and seemingly didn't care about *his* feelings. Yet she wasn't arrogant either, she was very respectful.

Her masculine energy did what it is meant to do: it defended and protected her. This mixture of the two energies is a very carefully crafted cocktail that can greatly serve any woman in the workplace and far beyond.

If you've ever seen the first season of the TV show *Suits*, then you've seen this concept of putting someone back in line. The show revolves around Harvey, a big-ass lawyer who believes he's the king of the world, and his intern Mike who's never afraid to stand up for himself. Harvey respects that a lot. If you don't stand up for yourself and what you believe in, nobody else will. And what you will notice is that although not everyone will respond favorably, most people will respect it a lot. Nobody respects a pushover.

The other party has two options: they can budge, which they will usually do. Or they can reject you, which will be good for you in the end as well. Never surround yourself with people who won't allow you to be you, as we've discussed.

Let's stay as far away from being a doormat as possible by making sure that you mix some masculine energy in when needed. "How do you know when it's needed?" you ask. That's what the next chapter is all about.

Do Not Negotiate with Terrorists

We must pick our battles. Had my sister's boss asked her to work late any other day, she probably would have. But given the importance of her weekend, this time it was non-negotiable. This battle was worth it, but I don't want to disguise that she worked really hard and was very flexible on many other occasions.

Boundaries that make you stick to your personal mission statement, to who you are, need to be protected with vigor.

But what happens when after stating your boundaries, someone decides to still walk across them as if they are nothing?

What if my sister's boss had told her to deal with it without listening to another word she said? That's what a toddler would do, so it was a possibility here.

The solution is that especially then, we stand our ground. I once heard someone from the state department explain an interesting concept. She dealt with kidnappings of citizens in foreign territories and spoke about a remarkable statistic. When experienced groups of terrorists or guerilla fighters kidnap a group of tourists to ask for ransom, they usually leave US citizens behind, alive and unharmed.

The US is a wealthy country, and US citizens are great targets, but the US is known for never negotiating with terrorists. It never pays ransom. Even the citizens who have been kidnapped in the past were later freed without paying ransom, according to that state official.

Why is this so important? If the US paid once, all bad guys all over the world would start kidnapping Americans because they would know they might get paid, even if it only happened sporadically. Americans would no longer be safe, anywhere.

When it *never* happens, there is no point.

When someone crosses your boundary and you let them, even if it's just once, there is no boundary. When the boss leaves after hearing your objection and returns on Monday to find you stood your ground, he'll know your boundaries are real the next time you state one.

This doesn't come without risks. You may get rejected, frowned upon, or suffer other consequences. Nevertheless, letting others walk over you is a whole lot worse in the long term.

Please keep in mind if you sporadically give in, you will create a huge precedent. You'll discover another reason why in the next chapter.

"This Isn't Like Me. Why Am I Doing This?"

This chapter deals with one of the most powerful psychological traps of them all. As soon as you set foot in it, you're stuck and your empowerment will vanish. This isn't just any trap; it will make you perform behaviors totally unlike you! You will literally start losing your mind to some extent. Most of the times you've caught yourself behaving in a way that was bad for you and unlike you, this trap was at play.

Enter the variable reward system. It is like the Bermuda triangle. When you come near the variable reward trap and you're unaware of it, your sanity will suddenly vanish.

You've seen the trap in action plenty of times. Ever wonder why some women stay with men who physically hit them? Or why they remain infatuated with a bad ex and cannot let go? Or why they continue working for a boss who keeps crossing their boundaries? Or why they keep hanging out with friends or family members who clearly don't care a single iota about them? It's because of this trap!

If bad men were to be bad 100% of the time, it would be easier to dump them and a lot fewer women would settle with one. The problem, however, is that these clowns show their good side every now and then, keeping that spark of hope alive that he *can* and will change one day.

If dead-end jobs hurt all the time, it would be easier to quit. When something good happens every now and then (e.g., the boss gives a compliment or a raise), it becomes easier to hope it will eventually get better.

Your mind tends to hang onto these positive moments and seems to forget about all the bad. And this too is not your fault,

139

as you'll learn.

B.F. Skinner, the scientist who taught pigeons how to play Ping-Pong, created something called a Skinner box. It's a simple box with a lever and a food-delivery system. Nothing fancy there, you'd think. Let's find out.

Skinner puts a pigeon in a box that gives food every time a lever is pushed. The pigeon walks around a bit and accidentally pushes the lever. Food comes out. The pigeon is stoked and does a little happy dance! Her worries are over, for now. A short while later, she's hungry again and pushes the same lever. Food comes out again.

Party time!

Our pigeon now knows how to ask for food at will, what a dream. She keeps pushing the lever and eats whenever she's hungry. Then, at some point, the food supply is empty. Pushing the bar no longer works. Not long after, the pigeon stops pushing. The party is over. She knows the lever won't do anything anymore, and she breaks up with her previous behavior. Nothing spectacular happened here.

For the second part of the experiment, Skinner redesigns the box a bit. When pushed, the lever now only gives food every so often. The delivery of food becomes variable. Shouldn't be a problem, right?

A different hungry pigeon enters the box. The pigeon walks around a bit and accidentally pushes the lever. Food comes out. The pigeon is stoked! Her worries are over. A short while later, she's hungry again and pushes the lever. This time, however, no food comes out. The pigeon's little brain is dazzled and wonders if the lever relieved her of her worries by giving her food earlier.

She recalls that it certainly did. So she pushes again. Food comes out this time.

Party time!

The pigeon sighs with relief; the lever still works.

A while later, the pigeon tries again. No food. She tries again. No food. Again. No food. Again. Food comes out. The pigeon's brain starts to short-circuit, and little clouds of steam are seen coming out of her ears. Her faith in the lever is gone because it is not consistent. Yet she did learn she shouldn't give up. As long as she keeps trying, food will come out eventually.

As I'm sure you can guess, the pigeon now frantically pushes the lever *all* the time. Seldom does food come, and she never knows when. When the food supply is truly gone, the pigeon keeps pushing frenziedly until she falls down from exhaustion.

This is the variable reward system in action. It gives a reward sporadically, and this is the very reason why you and I and all other humans frantically keep pushing the lever.

It's the scientifically proven reason why so many people keep scrolling down their social media feeds (pushing the lever) in the hopes of bumping upon a nice video, story, or picture that makes them feel good (the food). The dopamine response whenever it's party time is what keeps them hooked.[24]

This is the reason why so many women stay with men who treat them badly 90 percent of the time. They believe they have to keep trying and have to keep pushing the lever because they've seen firsthand there *is* some good in him (the 10 percent of the

---

[24] http://www.nirandfar.com/2012/03/want-to-hook-your-users-drive-them-crazy.html

time food is given).

The exact same system is at play in our professional lives, where some people may tend to accept a lot of BS as long as rewards are intermittently given.

And, as discussed in the previous chapter, this is the proof that explains why you must protect your boundaries *at all times*. When you allow sporadic crossings, others will keep marching over in a frenzy.

If you tell a kid he can't do something ten times but fold the eleventh time he asks, he will keep asking because he has now learned you will budge at some point in time. He just needs to try long enough. It's a trap and a devious one, especially when you're on the receiving end.

The solution is simple. See the trap for what it is and become aware of it.

When you sense that you accept bad behavior from anyone and are unsure why, ask yourself, "Am I acting like that pigeon? Am I stuck in the variable reward system here? Is someone giving me sporadic treats to hook me up and make me lose my sanity?"

As soon as you sense the trap is at play or you realize you've been treated badly but are sticking around for the leftovers you seldom get, it's time to get out of the box! This awareness is all it takes to realign your behavior.

Fortunately, this is not the only box that counts.

The Big Box of Stuff

Your identity is defined by what your response is to the "who am I?" question. Your identity stands for everything you currently are and have in your life. Not your material belongings but what you spend time and energy upon, what you worry about, what makes you happy, what moves and touches you.

The identity of a 23-year-old woman could be, "I'm passionate about history, and I'm studying to become a history teacher. I love spending time with my friends. I travel a lot, and my family is very important to me. I also love jogging, working out, and eating healthy. I'm a vegan too. I hate harming animals."

A 30-year-old woman may say, "I'm a sales representative, and I'm good at it. I like my colleagues, just not Bob; he's always staring at me. I'm also the wife of Peter, a great guy who works as a delivery courier. I'm the mother of Sasha and Flynn whom I adore very much. I take good care of them and make sure I give them a good upbringing. I don't have time for much else besides my family."

A 60-year-old woman's identity can be, "I love taking long walks on the beach with Fido, my husband. I enjoy having the grandchildren over, but I do love the quiet moments as well. I try to stay active and am passionate about yoga. I lead a team of twenty-three people at work and love doing it."

That's who these women currently are.

The importance of your identity is not to be underestimated. People who lose their identity get depressed, burnt out, and will generally feel bad for a long time. That's logical since they no longer know who they are or what they stand for. They are purposeless, mission-less, and adrift in life.

This can happen to a woman who sees her kids leave for college and has a hard time adapting to her new role in the now empty house. The couple that was in an interdependent relationship until the break-up or everyone else who experiences a big change in life.

In other words, you need to build your identity upon the right foundation, not on quicksand. Otherwise, it becomes easy to lose yourself.

Your life is built upon loads of little elements. Consider your life a big box with a fixed size. You cannot enlarge the box. All of the aspects of your life are in that box. Ideally, you'd fill it with loads of little to medium-sized items like work life and going to the gym. There would be elements for your friends, pets, children, your different hobbies, spending time watching your favorite TV show, going for a nice meal with friends, and so on. Loads of different elements that, when placed out on the table, wouldn't vary a lot in size.

That's the ideal, balanced situation where your identity is built upon these practically same-sized components.

Suppose that's the case, and the element that represents your job falls away. Would that change your identity? Probably not. It's only a small part of the big puzzle. Or what if the piece that stands for your relationship is removed? Would that change your identity? No, not really; there are plenty of other puzzle pieces still left in the box.

This is not to say you wouldn't miss that component of your life, that you wouldn't mourn the loss for a while, but your identity— who you are in your core—wouldn't change.

Now consider a different type of woman. Ever since she left high school, she's been a high achiever. If you looked into her box, your eyes would immediately be drawn to the huge *job* and one medium-sized *relationship* pieces. The little crumbles at the bottom of the box representing her friendships, hobbies, and more are *so* small, you would probably not even notice them at all. All she does is work, read magazines about success, have power lunches with powerful people, invite important people over for dinner, and spend some time with the hubby during the weekends mostly still talking about business. That's it!

Imagine this woman gets to hear the most ridiculously worded phrase in the world, "I'm sorry, but we will have to let you go" as if they are doing her a favor. The huge job component is suddenly removed from the box. No warning was given. She hadn't seen it coming. Do you think this would hurt her identity?

You bet! It's smashed into smithereens overnight!

If this woman doesn't find a similar job (similar pay, similar responsibilities, similar recognition from the outside world) pronto, she will collapse and fall to pieces within a week or two. You'll need a broom and a dustpan to clean her up.

This woman will no longer know how to behave toward the few friends she has. She'll be afraid to hear "how's it going?" from the Joneses next door. She will undoubtedly recluse herself. Why wouldn't she? Who is she going to invite for dinner now? And what will they talk about?

She's lost.

I'm sure it's clear why. Her job was *everything*, and her life box only had so many other items on the inside. Almost all of her eggs were in two baskets; the rest was made up of crumbles.

When you build your life upon two pillars, trouble will occur as soon as there's a problem with one of those supports. It's impossible not to tumble down upon removing one of them.

First of all, having just a couple of pillars makes you needy. When all of your life juice comes from one or two sources, you will invest a lot of your time and energy into it. You become dependent.

Women, much more than men, need a sense of community, as previously discussed. The workaholic in the example tries to tap into community from networking and power lunches, but these will only give her a fraction of the real sense of friendship she needs. It's not a surrogate for the real thing, for real relationships. And that's just one example of the many items that are missing.

The second challenge in this case is that deep down you already know your identity is built on shaky ground. It will never feel safe and secure; like you're standing on an unstable ladder. Even though you keep climbing, the instability only increases. These are the people who lie awake at night, afraid they might lose it all. They might since they have so little in their life box.

What about your box?

Take a piece of paper, and draw all of the items you have in your life. How big are they? You'll *see* what may have grown out of proportion and what other boxes you may need to introduce.

This is a personal challenge for me too. I tend to naturally put most of my time and energy in the "entrepreneur" element. That's the biggest one for me, second is my relationship, and then there's not a lot of time left for everything else. I've always been like that ever since I was a kid. But lately, I've learned to consciously decide what other elements I should grow because, and here's the kicker, they will actually help my two most important pillars.

By spending more time and energy on other items like friends, working out, eating healthy, listening to music, the size of my most important pieces—my business and my relationship—will decrease, but the *quality* of those boxes will increase! That's very counterintuitive and why so many people have a hard time coping with it.

If all of your time is spent on your relationship, I can assure you it won't be a good one. If all of your energy is spent on working, your productivity will plummet and your health will suffer greatly. If all of your time is allotted to raising kids, your health and relationship will suffer from an ever-growing sensation of frustration.

When I take time to go for a thirty- or even sixty-minute walk, my productivity is much higher afterward, and my business benefits. When I spend time with friends, I'm happy to return home and see my girlfriend whereas I wouldn't have noticed how much I missed her had I spent every moment *with* her.

The goal of this chapter is to simply plant a little seed and have you draw out your life's boxes. If you see most or your time is spent on just a few elements, what are other areas you *should* spend more time on but haven't been doing so? Put more time into those additional aspects of your life for thirty days, even and especially when you believe you don't have time for it.

Thirty days. It's just a test.

Then come back to the drawing board and analyze what has

changed. Go from there and decide what other elements deserve more of your time and energy going forward.

As the weeks pass, you will feel your identity strengthening and your pure confidence growing. The quicksand will start to disappear, and you will feel a stability that you may have been missing out on for a long time.

Certain worries will vanish, fears will disappear, and it will be a lot easier to be strict about your boundaries because *if* you're ever let go by a job or a man, it won't be *that* big of a deal. Your identity will remain intact, and you will bounce back quicker.

"Never Show Your Back. And Whatever You Do, Don't Run!"

I've had my fair share of walks in the wilderness. And each and every time the guide advised, "If you do see a wild predator, don't turn your back to it! Whatever you do, never turn your back to it. Never run. Slowly step aside or withdraw, but never run or show your back. If the animal does come for you, make yourself as big as possible and yell with the loudest voice with the most bass you can bear."

"Great," I thought. "I already run and scream like a little boy when I see a spider, but when I'm face-to-face with an angry bear I'm supposed to act calm, cool, and collected? That will be fun..."

That made me wonder why you shouldn't show your back when you meet a lion or a bear or any other predator for that matter. It turns out that simple move makes you the prey and that wild animal the predator. The predator has a built-in instinct that states, "If it runs away and turns its back to me, it's afraid. So then I *can and should* eat it." Simple.

If, however, you keep looking at the animal and don't run or turn your back, it will gauge you and try to figure out who's who. The predator isn't sure yet. For all it knows, you may be poisonous or have some sharp teeth and the capacity to devour it in seconds.

I've luckily never had to practice this strategy, but I've heard stories from people who have. And it worked. One guy was able to stop a roaring lion that was running toward him. And a clip on YouTube shows[25] a man who angers an elephant that starts to storm toward him. This guy, laughing and truly unaware of the

---

[25] https://www.youtube.com/watch?v=1b-WaWMaze0

149

danger, stands still and shows the stop sign with his hand. Can you imagine? The elephant stops indeed, inches before hitting the dumbfounded tourist. The elephant had been bluffing and preferred not to risk a fight since "if that little man doesn't run, he's either really stupid or superbly powerful."

Showing fear or running away makes you the prey.

This is not a book about wandering around in the wilderness. Or is it? I believe this to be a nice analogy for life as a whole. There are predators everywhere! Horrible bosses, nasty competitors, backstabbing friends. Need I go on?

When you fear what other people think of you, some will take advantage of it. Bullies will find you either way and even good people will push your hot buttons to manipulate your actions.

Have you ever noticed how some people are good at spotting your weaknesses only to then exploit them by pointing them out over and over again? Or how some people try to impose upon you? Some are really good at this in the workplace. They like to act and feel important and are looking for prey, people they can dominate. They feed upon it; it's the only way they can raise their own fake self-esteem. As they push other people down, they believe theirs goes up.

If that ever happens, don't show your back. Show them that you're not the prey, and then devour *them* in seconds.

Here are some ways to make this happen:

- When you don't want to comply, do not make it open to debate. Never ask if the other person agrees after making an assertive statement. The other party shouldn't feel you're hoping they will be fine with it. Their opinion does not matter! Lay down the law—your law. If they don't agree, they can turn their backs to you.

I'm making it sound harsh, but it isn't. There is no arrogance involved. I would like to point to the example of my sister again. Laying down her law is exactly what she did. She wasn't arrogant or weak. Never ask if the manipulators agree. Of course, they don't!

Some people who try to state their boundaries are *still* seeking the approval of others. They might say, "I can't do that. I hope you understand." That's weakness because it proves you're still trying to gain their approval. If it's one of your boundaries, the opinions of others don't matter. It's not a negotiation.

- When someone makes a stupid remark, one intended to hurt you or to put you off balance, ask him/her to repeat it. This is simple, just calmly say, "What did you just say to me?" and then stop talking. Allow the silence to be as long as required. Having the others repeat it forces *them* to explain themselves and think about what they just said or did.

  This is a major power shift that turns the predator into the prey. They think they're coming from a position of strength, but their attack bounces off of you and goes straight back to them *without* you becoming emotional or showing in any way that they've gotten to you.

- When someone acted like a manipulator in the past and tried to hurt you in any way, don't let them emotionally near again. If it was on purpose, they will do it again. And sure, you can fend it off, but as we've learned, the people that surround you influence you heavily. They'd better not be predators, or you will always have to sleep with one eye open.

- Watch out whenever you're doing something against your will. Other people have unique ways to manipulate us. A family member of mine knew I didn't want to be "selfish," so whenever she wanted to change my behavior she told me I was acting selfishly. If you do realize someone got you to do something that you would normally have declined, have a look at what they said or did to change your mind. That's often their modus operandi, and they will use it again. This time, however, you'll see it coming.

In conclusion, never behave like the prey.

The Power of Vulnerability

Just about everyone is attracted to authentic people, people who don't play a role, people who don't wear a mask, people who are confident in their uniqueness and are not afraid to show it to the world.

As humans, people tend to mistrust others who show them one image of themselves and another image to someone else. People have very intelligent B.S. radars and generally dislike and don't trust people who wear masks.

Another reason that people who hide behind masks are repulsive is because they portray weakness. Someone who wears a figurative mask is trying to either cover up pure badness or pure weakness. It's never used to cover up greatness.

Here's why vulnerability and not shielding your uniqueness is powerful. Please take a moment to imagine an arena with two gladiators. Gladiator number one is unexperienced and new, has a shield, and he's frantically hiding behind it. He makes himself as small as possible and uses his hands to protect vital organs. The public hears a subtle "mommy" resounding from behind the shield. Gladiator number two has been around for a while, is standing without a shield but has a big grin on his face. He holds his head up high and has his chest forward. He's not even wearing a helmet!

If I would ask you who the most powerful gladiator is, which one would you pick?

It will probably not be the one calling for his mommy. The gladiator without a shield is the stronger one. It seems like he has less fear or even no fear whatsoever. He's either an idiot who's about to be chopped into little pieces, or he must be really powerful. But the fact that he's still a gladiator with all limbs attached proves he must be quite good; otherwise, he would have been eliminated a long time ago.

Now, why is he so powerful? He hasn't even fought yet! It's because he's vulnerable. His chest, containing his most important organs like his heart, is unprotected. His head, containing the few brain cells every man has, is exposed. So he *must* be powerful. The weakling hiding behind his shield, trying to protect everything, is clearly not confident that he will win this fight. The one who is vulnerable emits a lot of power.

Having the guts to show your vulnerability is powerful, as counterintuitive as that may sound.

The weakest animals crawl and hide, with their tails between their legs and ears down, trying to make themselves as small as possible. The strong animals, however, walk proudly and are exposed. They're neither hiding nor protecting themselves. They may just be legends in their own minds, but you won't consider them weaklings.

During my research of the high-value women and my more than a decade of coaching women, I noticed that some women are afraid to be vulnerable. They want everything to be under control and continuously look for certainty. They feel needy in their relationships, insecure in their job functions, and they're perpetually hiding behind a variety of shields in an effort to never get hurt.

Now as we've seen, it's impossible to not get hurt. And you don't win a fight by hiding either. The women who were not afraid to get a punch, to fall down, to lose, to fail, and to get hurt had much fuller lives and, most importantly, were hurt less!

Allow me to use relationships as an example again, because that's something everyone has experience with.

Here's a little pop-quiz. Who will get hurt the most?

Woman A is fearful and needy. She is trying to make sure no one can hurt her, so she needs to know where "this" is going and how fast it is moving there. Of course! She wants to make sure her boyfriend will eventually ask her to marry him, and she wants to get rid of her feelings of insecurity from not knowing. So she asks him often. Woman A needs confirmation that all will be fine, all the time.

She knows it's wrong to behave like that, so she tries to play a normal and secure woman. Nevertheless every now and then her true personality shines through the cracks of her mask, especially when she breaks down in a neediness frenzy, when she cries a bit, sulks a bit, and says things like, "I'm not sure that you love me as much as I love you" while wiping off the tears on her face. She frantically avoids getting hurt, yet she feels hurt all the time.

I'm sure I don't even need to explain who Woman B is for you to know where this is going, but let's have at it. Woman B also wants to get married to a good guy. Her boyfriend seems like a good man; otherwise, she wouldn't be with him. She has decided she's not going to bring up a possible marriage. She has bouts of neediness and worry too, but she dismisses them and doesn't try to make them go away by seeking out reassurance. She knows he might eventually not marry her and turn out to be a player or a bad boy, but she doesn't care. *If* she gets hurt, so be it, she wants to enjoy the great moments they have together. She'll deal with the hurt when it comes, *not beforehand*.

If this is the way both relationships progress, guess what woman will have the highest probability of getting hurt and *not* getting married in the end? Woman A. It's a self-fulfilling prophecy. Woman B might get hurt, but because she's vulnerable she has much more fun in life in general.

True power comes from being vulnerable and dealing with hurt as it comes, never beforehand.

It's much easier to be confident and go for what you want both on a personal and a professional level when you're OK with being vulnerable. Most importantly, it's much easier to be authentic!

"Easier said than done, Brian" is what I often hear. And sure, it is! If it were easy, every person would be a high-value woman or man.

Arianna Huffington, the high-value woman who founded *The Huffington Post*, once gave the advice that women should allow themselves to be emotional (to be vulnerable), to even react emotionally, to feel anger and sadness ... and to then move on. Not fighting your emotions is one of the most important secrets I've ever discovered. Allow, accept, and move on.

But the deeper message I'm trying to pass along here is that *if you want to be fully empowered, you cannot shield off your flaws.*

Show them! Don't hide. It's a remarkable sign of strength and self-confidence. Don't ever feel ashamed about all that you are *not*. It's what makes you unique. And again, showing your weaknesses *is* a sign of strength. Other people respect that so much more than wearing a mask or covering up.

Imagine a work meeting. You have an important position, and you're sitting at the head of the table. You ask Woman A, "Can you tell me the best strategy to get our 10 percent growth next quarter?" The woman, totally flabbergasted by the question, responds, "Um, well, I would do a bit of this and a bit of that, and then..." trying to come across as well educated on the subject.

Asked the exact same question, Woman B handles it differently. She says, "Yes, but I'll get back to you on that. There are some numbers I don't know by heart that I want to check first." She has just shown a major flaw: she's not an encyclopedia that knows everything about everything.

Guess which woman will be respected, paid, and appreciated the most? Woman B has just shown you can trust her, she won't make anything up to please you, she doesn't pretend. She's her authentic, mask-less, take-it-or-leave-it self.

Vulnerability and having the figurative balls to show your flaws are signs of strength.

Turning Princes into Frogs

As you move forward and push the pedal of your empowerment engine to the metal, you'll have to be careful with the men in your life. Men are very sensitive creatures, given their delicate egos, and may start to act in weird ways when you let out your lioness. Be careful that you don't emasculate the men around you, especially not the man you're in love with since you might accidentally turn your prince into a frog.

If women ask men to tone it down, be more considerate, have more empathy, or treat them better *when these men already give it all they've got...* these women will start to see strange behavior because they are actually castrating those men and asking them to not be one. I want to reiterate that I'm talking about men who are doing the best they can.

This can then go two ways. He may become an approval-seeking wussy and try to adapt to the whims of the dominatrix he's with. Most women get fed up with guys like these in less than one date. They often love a good foot massage, but when their guy starts kissing their feet relentlessly, they will lose interest quickly.

Or, and this is often even worse, the man will fear getting intimate with his woman. Not just between the bed sheets but in the relationship as a whole. He'll become so distant and cautious that you may start to wonder where he went. His body is still there, yet his behavior resembles that of a shy little boy. If you're married, then you'll see him hanging out in the garage more often, fiddling with his tools, or God knows what else. Or he may start to come home from work later and later because he's afraid of what he'll be "punished" for when he arrives home.

When you castrate a man, one of the other unwanted behaviors you'll see is jealousy, and not just toward the other men in your life. If you get a raise or reach another goal, he will not like it. Everything will start to feel like a competition to him.

Castrating a man gives him two options. He can compete with you, or kneel and treat you like a goddess. Either way, you lose because his feelings will transform from attraction to fear.

So how do you prevent this? Because you should never put a limit on your own empowerment. You don't need to tone it down either.

It's simple. We've seen that the primary mission for men is to provide for and protect the woman they love. They want to be important to her. Some women inadvertently weaken him by taking that important mission away from their man.

Here are some examples:

- "I don't need your help. I can change that lamp on my own, thank you very much."
- "Thanks, but no, I don't want you to pay for dinner. I can pay for my own food. I'm a grown-up, and we're no longer living in the fifties, are we?"
- "Did you hear John, Marie's husband, got a big promotion? He's so successful. So how was your day today?"
- "The Jeffersons have booked a vacation to Hawaii. They take more vacations than we do!"

These are all examples of attacking his manhood. Some may not make any sense to you, as a woman. What you'll notice, however, is that every sentence communicates: "I don't need you and/or I'm not happy with the way you take care of me. You're not as good as other men."

I never said men were insensitive.

When a man feels that he's not good enough for you, especially when you're communicating it to him, he cannot be your prince. He will feel like a frog.

That's why it is excruciatingly important to never try to change your man by complaining or nagging. He will feel like a loser and will start acting like one. That's quite logical when he hears sentences like:

- "Why don't you ever…"
- "Why aren't you like Mike, Janie's husband, who…"
- "I feel like you no longer love me" (even though he's *really* doing the best he can in this case. We're still working under the premise that in these examples the man you're with is a good one who's giving it all he's got).

Never underestimate the sensitivity of a man's ego. All these sentences are communicating that he's not man enough for you. That's pure castration!

If he truly loves you, all he wants to do is take care of you, give you what you need, regardless of how successful you are. But you won't get there by castrating him. He'll think, "What's the point anyway? It's clear I can't make her happy so I might as well stop trying."

If you want to change his behavior, there are better ways than castration or placing blame. Simply give him compliments when he's showing behavior you want to enforce and *ignore him* whenever he does something you don't like.

Say this:

- "I love it how you take out the trash, honey. That's one thing less for me to worry about."
- "I see you drank less beer this week. That's great! I think I'm starting to see your six pack abs coming back!"
- "Thanks for cooking, honey. It makes me proud to be with a man who knows his way around the kitchen."

Instead of:

- "Do you *really* need another beer?"
- "For once in your life could you make dinner for yourself instead of relying on me every night?"
- "Why don't you ever take out the trash? I mean, I'm already worrying about everything else around here. It's the ONLY thing I ask of you." [Ask it once, kindly, then let the trash pile up until he does it out of his own will. When he finally does (he will!), give a compliment. Then you'll see him do more of it. Whatever works on raising a puppy or a three-year-old will work on men. (Trust me, I'm one of them.)]

On the other hand, if you ever *really* want to hurt a man, just attack his manhood by telling him he's not enough of a man. That will be more painful to him than scratching the paint of his car or hiding the TV-remote (both horrendous events for men).

I'll explain what happens inside his mind when you make him feel like a man, but I'll have to bring on the strippers first...

What Do Strippers Have to Do with Anything?

I went to Vegas many years ago when a good friend of mine got married. As I walked into a strip club with a group of guys, we each had a lovely woman join us. I admit that was a magical moment; my prayers had finally been answered.

First of all, that never happens in real life. Even the best-looking men don't enter a club and then automatically have a pretty woman walk up to them, grab them by the arm, and ask how their day is going.

This was *manipulator* strategy number one of the stripper. Everything that happens in the strip club is carefully orchestrated to make men feel like they are not only legends in their own minds but in her mind as well. Even though rationally we all knew these strippers weren't interested in our riveting personalities, it worked.

My stripper, Bella, explained it was her first night in the joint. Recently moved from Los Angeles and still a bit insecure was her story. This, although it turned out to be true, was *manipulator* strategy number two—the damsel in distress, taking advantage of men wanting to provide and protect.

Lovely Bella then started to compliment me and say things like:
- "You're so handsome."
- "Oh, it must not have been easy to achieve this and that."
- "You must be really important."

Mind you, these were not reactions to me trying to show off, I was just thinking about gnomes and squirrels in order to not get under her spell.

Between us, even though I knew it was all as fake as Santa Claus (and I even made that absolutely clear to her), it was working. The lion inside me started to roar. I felt my masculine energy flourishing as she was pushing all of the right buttons.

When a woman *figuratively* nurtures a man's manhood, it feels like heaven.

When he loves that woman, all heaven breaks loose. There is no greater feeling to any man than to know that the woman he loves sees him as the *best man* out there. I call this ego feeding. When a woman helps a man to be all the man he can be, the clouds disappear and the birds of happiness start to sing on his shoulders. In turn, every good man will help you become the woman you can be too. That goes without saying.

When you get to that place, which is the opposite of male-castration, he will no longer see you as competition, regardless of how successful you are compared to him.

When was the last time you shared how impressed you were by what an important man in your life had done? It doesn't have to be a lover; it can be a male colleague or even a good friend.

See what it does to his energy and his eyes when you give a sincere compliment.

One word of caution, compliments and praise should never be given from a position of weakness and neediness. The stripper wanted some of my money, but she wasn't needy. She was in control at all times. If I hadn't given her attention, she would have moved over to the next lap. She never needed me. That's why it worked.

If you are more successful than the man you're in a relationship with, just make sure he still feels he's important to you. You can say things like, "I love it how I can discuss business ideas with you. I love your insights" or "I love it how you take care of me. It allows me to operate at my best at work." That's all his ego will need. I've coached many very successful women who had castration-problems in their relationships. Letting him know he's still important to you is all he needs to know.

This works on all men. You can use it whenever you want to make a man feel good for whatever reason.

Men always live for becoming the hero.

Our Souls Never Give Up

As you are nearing the end of this book and are thinking about the changes that may need to be made in your life, you may start to feel frustrated. You may wish you had taken different paths in the past or, as some women wrote in their reviews of my other books, "If only I had known this earlier!"

I have good news for you: our soul never gives up. It continues to grow until the day we leave this Earth.

It never ceases to amaze me how plants respond to getting trimmed. When you cut off a twig, the remaining twig will split and form multiple new branches. When you cut those, each and every one of those twigs will multiply as well. You can trim the bushes as much as you want; as long as the soul, the purpose of the plant stays alive, it's never ever going to give up. As long as you don't remove the roots from the ground or poison the plant with pesticides, it will keep adapting and will keep trying to fulfill its mission.

So do we.

Whatever it is you got wrong in the past, there is always time to make it right. Your past can still be accepted, treasured, and learned from. You don't choose the obstacles and problems you face, but you do always choose your attitude.

Plus, in my opinion, mistakes and bad choices are good. I strongly believe in the saying, "What doesn't kill us makes us stronger." Every so-called failure is just information. True failure only occurs when you stop trying and quit.

Just as hurt cannot be avoided, making mistakes can't be either. The more successful the person, the more spectacular the mistakes she or he will have made in the past. They chose to not be ashamed of those mistakes, to not critique themselves for making them, to learn from them, and to then let them go.

Thomas Edison, the guy who invented the light bulb who struggled massively when making his discovery, is known for saying, "I have not failed. I just found 10,000 ways that won't work."

The secret to life is a positive attitude. You have one, I have one, we all have one. *Regardless* of what is happening to us! Everyone was born with a positive attitude.

The south of the United States has had their fair share of flooding and storms in the last twenty years. And it happened again not so long ago. As I was watching news coverage of the event, an elderly couple was being interviewed. They were sitting on a bus on the tarmac of the airport, waiting for the army plane that would get them out of there. After they had been evacuated from their home because of the rising water, they were told it would be impossible to return in the first couple of weeks. On top of that, everything was probably lost anyway. When floodwater enters a home and sits there for more than a day at high temperatures, the house becomes a breeding nest of molds, bacteria, and other toxins.

All of their belongings had been left at the flooded house. Yet here they were, Mr. and Mrs. Smith, sitting on the bus with huge grins on their faces, excited for the journey ahead of them. The journalist found that a strange sight since most of the people he had previously interviewed were crying.

"Well, I just got the test results back last week," Mrs. Smith said. "I had breast cancer, and I survived it. The cancer is gone for now!"

"But you just lost your house and all of your belongings. Doesn't that make you sad?" the puzzled journalist asked.

"No of course not! We're lucky! I'm sitting here alive! And my husband just had his hip replaced."

The journalist and the camera turned to the husband who's still grinning like a kid visiting Santa. I'm not exaggerating.

"Aren't *you* sad?" the journalist asked.

"Sad? Why would I be sad? What good would it do if you would go through life feeling sad and being negative?"

Amazing.

This is the true power that the likes of Roman Emperor Marcus Aurelius, the captured Jewish doctor Viktor Frankl, the South African president Nelson Mandela, former First Lady Michelle Obama, and so many other high-value people have been using day in and day out.

Your soul wants to be positive, and it will never give up.

And She Lives Happily Ever After... or Does She?

Don't you love how every chick flick ends with the heroine and the hero falling in love and sailing off into the totally certain future of unconditional love and never-ending blissful happiness? How many real people do you know like that? Chances are not a lot ... maybe none.

Everyone has their problems, and good times never last forever. Love is not unconditional, and the prince on the white horse does not exist.

The actor Robert Redford once told *Esquire Magazine*: "Life is essentially sad. Happiness is sporadic. It comes in moments, and that's it. Extract the blood from every moment."[26]

As you've seen throughout the book, high-value people don't fight any of it. They don't look for perpetual happiness but thoroughly enjoy the moments whenever they come. I believe that to be a very important phenomenon because I can honestly say that I've ruined many happy moments while worrying about challenges that never even manifested. My life used to be a constant struggle, and I forgot to enjoy the moments I could have been happy. High-value people have taught me it's fine to let go every now and then, to go with the flow. When you feel down, accept it and move on. When you feel happy, enjoy it and move on.

This is where the high-value woman finds her strength. She's never needy and manages her emotions pretty well because she sees right through them. She's living *her* life. She focuses on what's important to her. Even though she hopes to find a lot of

---

[26] http://www.esquire.com/entertainment/interviews/a9133/robert-redford-quotes-0111/

moments of blissful happiness, a great guy to grow old with, a pristine health report, all of these are not a must. It's not a need. She's totally fulfilled either way because she chooses to.

She comes first.

Final Words

Thank you for reading this book and for making it until the end. I hope you found it inspiring. I've loved writing it for you. I've spent years researching these topics and coaching women to get the results the high-value woman successfully achieves. I hope you'll use what I've described. You deserve the results that go with it!

If you didn't like the book, please reach out to me on brian@briannox.com. I value your feedback.

Did you like it? I sincerely hope so. Then please share your thoughts on Amazon so other women just like you can find out more about the book and what it meant to you. Reviewing is easy. Go to the book by typing in the title in Amazon, scroll down to the review section, and click on "Write a customer review." You have my eternal gratitude.

Thanks for reading!

Brian

P.S. **And if you want even more tips and strategies**, sign up for my FREE advanced tactics newsletter on shecomesfirstbook.com and join the large group of women who already receive it.

More Books by Brian Nox:

- Enough! How to stop feeling overwhelmed

- F*ck Him! Nice Girls Always Finish Single

- Red Flags: How to know he's playing games with you

- Are You Scaring Him Away?

- 21 Traps You need to avoid in Dating & Relationships

Made in the USA
Columbia, SC
29 February 2020